T

Healthy Skin

A Lifetime Guide to Beautiful, Problem-Free Skin

Lynn J. Parentini

PRENTICE HALL
Englewood Cliffs, NJ 07632

Prentice Hall International (UK) Limited, *London*
Prentice Hall of Australia Pty. Limited, *Sydney*
Prentice Hall Canada, Inc., *Toronto*
Prentice Hall Hispanoamericana, S.A., *Mexico*
Prentice Hall of India Private Limited, *New Delhi*
Prentice Hall of Japan, Inc., *Tokyo*
Simon & Schuster Asia Pte. Ltd., *Singapore*
Editora Prentice Hall do Brasil, Ltda., *Rio de Janeiro*

10 9 8 7 6 5 4 3 2 1

Library of Congress Cataloging in Publication Data

Parentini, Lynn.
The joy of healthy skin / Lynn Parentini.
p. cm.
Includes index.
ISBN 0-13-127267-5 (cloth). — ISBN 0-13-127275-6 (pbk.)
1. Skin—Care and hygiene. I. Title.
RL85.P365 1995
646.7'26—dc20 95-37691
CIP

ISBN 0-13-127267-5 (C)
ISBN 0-13-127275-6 (P)

PRENTICE HALL
Englewood Cliffs, NJ 07632

A Simon & Schuster Company

Printed in the United States of America

I would like to dedicate this book to my late beloved grandmother Mildred, who taught me in her 100+ years, that you have to be like a willow tree in life and bend with life's vicissitudes.

To my grandmother Francis, who's pragmatic approach to life has had such a profound and positive effect on me in meeting life's challenges.

To the memory of Alfred M. Golish, who gave me my start in Corporate America, and whose generosity and humor has had such an indelible impression on me. I am forever grateful to him.

To my stepdaughter Jamie Schwartz-Ritter, thank you for helping me with some of the leg work.

Mom and Dad, thank you for all your moral support.

ACKNOWLEDGMENTS

To my dear husband and best friend Harvey Schwartz thank you for all your extra love and support while writing this book.

To my daughter Dana, a very special thank you for always being there for me.

A big thank you to my entire family (the Parentini, Schwartz, DeCara, Cavalluzzi, Bianchi, and Arrighi clan) for all the moral support.

To my dearest friend Dolores, thank you for all your great typing skills.

To Denise Jacob of the American Academy of Dermatology and Lisa Kamen of the American Academy of Cosmetic Surgery thank you for supplying me with the most current statistics and medical options for skin cancer.

Special thanks to Bianca Steinle and Marco Mongillo for bringing publisher and author together.

Grateful acknowledgment is also made to the following for permission to reprint previously published material:

American Academy of Dermatology, illustration on p. 8 and press releases on pp. 266-270.

American College of Cosmetic Surgery, descriptions of cosmetic surgical procedures on pp. 285-307.

Canyon Ranch, recipes on pp. 103-114 and photograph on p. 311.

Four Seasons Resort and Club, recipes on pp. 136-143 and photograph on p. 153.

PGA National Resort and Spa, recipes on pp. 114-136 and photograph on p. 312.

Spa Grande at the Grand Wailea Resort, photograph on p. 316.

Terme di Saturnia, Tuscany Region, Italy, photograph on pp. 324, 326.

Thalassotherapy/The Seawater Thermal Bath of Monte Carlo, photograph on p. 323.

The Oriental Spa Thai Health and Beauty Center, Bangkok, Thailand, photograph on p. 148.

The Spa Internazionale at Fisher Island Club, photograph on p. 333.

Lynn J. Parentini

Introduction

Did you know there is a "secret beauty regime" that will make your skin look young and healthy? You will truly be surprised just how easy it is to achieve a healthier complexion when you open *The Joy of Healthy Skin.* This book was designed to be a "complete source" of skin care, with emphasis on both corrective and preventive care. Most importantly, the information provided can be used with any skin product and be applied to any skin type, problem, or immediate need.

Each page of this book will present to you an accurate picture of skin care, from products to ingredients to medical options that will show you how to care for your skin with each of your successive life stages.

The Joy of Healthy Skin has been divided into three special sections. Part One, "Beauty At Home," teaches you all the details you need to care for your skin in a practical and cost-effective manner. Learn the latest head-to-toe home care beauty recipes that will help your complexion glow with health. Part Two, "Special Considerations," focuses on everything you wanted to know about different situations that could cause skin problems and premature aging. Here you will discover a full spectrum of straight-to-the point nutritional advice that will have a positive impact on your complexion. Finally, Part Three, "Professional Care," taps into the latest dermatology, cosmetic surgery, and esthetic technology resources and treatments available to you. This section features advice from world-renowned, board-certified dermatologists and cosmetic surgeons.

Learn the latest up-to-date facts, anti-aging procedures, and advice on how to keep your skin as young as it can be. You will also discover valuable advice from leading estheticians and spa experts from famous spas around the U.S. and the world.

This book will put you in the driver's seat by increasing your awareness so you can intelligently care for and protect your skin. You can participate in my unique skin tests, all of which will teach you exactly what you need to do for your skin at all times. Quiz yourself with "Eighteen Ways to Identify Your Skin Type," "Nine Ways to Test Your Skin for Sensitivities" (both found in Chapter Two), and "Seven Ways to Test Your Sun Knowledge" (located in Chapter Ten).

Spectacular results can be achieved with very little skin care maintenance. You can reveal a fresher, and even a younger, more radiant looking skin in no time at all. Be your skin's best friend by following the hundreds of "Age Busting" and "Healthful" tips that will keep your skin in tip-top shape. Learn how you can smooth away years of skin abuse with simple, over-the-counter products, special vitamin and mineral supplements, and with a unique category of power foods for your skin.

This practical approach to skin care will help you discover scores of no-nonsense home remedies, at-home beauty prescriptions, anti-aging treatments, valuable skin-saving bits of advice, precautions that could save you from disastrous skin problems, and plenty of sensible skin tips, all of which will become your personal "Lifetime Guide to Beautiful, Problem-Free Skin."

Contents

Chapter Two

TAKE CONTROL LEARN HOW TO RECOGNIZE YOUR SKIN TYPE AND CONDITION

Chapter Three

THE NO-NONSENSE SKIN-CARE PROGRAM THAT FITS ANY BUSY LIFESTYLE 43

Chapter Four

FEEDING YOUR SKIN FROM WITHIN

Chapter Five

TURN YOUR HOME INTO A SPA FOR THE WEEKEND 145

Chapter Six

CREATE AN AROMATHERAPY BEAUTY OASIS AT HOME 173

PART TWO
Special Considerations

Chapter Seven
JUST FOR MEN

Chapter Eight
SEASONAL SKIN CARE

Chapter Nine

TIMELESS BEAUTY
UNDERSTANDING THE DYNAMICS OF CARING FOR MATURE SKIN
227

Chapter Ten

TANNING—THE GOOD AND THE BAD 253

Chapter Eleven

BEAUTY ON THE ROAD MADE SIMPLE
275

PART THREE
Professional Care
281

Chapter Twelve

MEDICAL UPDATE! DERMATOLOGY AND COSMETIC SURGERY OPTIONS
283

Chapter Fourteen

DISCOVER THE TRADE SECRETS OF LEADING ESTHETICIANS AND SPA EXPERTS
335

Appendix A

THE ABCs OF SKIN-CARE PRODUCTS
351

Appendix B

SOURCES OF INFORMATION FOR YOUR SKIN
355

Index

357

Part ONE

Beauty at Home

CHAPTER *One*

THE SKIN! WHAT MAKES IT TICK

Myths and old wives' tales abound about the largest organ of the body—the skin. It's these persistent falsehoods, mixed in through the years with reams of scientific facts and findings that make day-to-day, at-home skin care so confusing. That's why I've written this book. I want to put an end to the myths, share some factual tidbits, and personally guide you through the ins and outs of skin-care management.

In this first chapter, we'll take a look at the structure and function of the skin. It's easier to intelligently care for your skin if you understand what makes it work. There are libraries containing hundreds of medical books that scientifically explore the skin. So, of course, it's impossible to tell you everything there is to know in one short chapter. But I can highlight the most important points and add some bits of interesting trivia about the most unique wonders and truths of the skin.

SKIN CARE TRIVIA . . . SIX FUN FACTS

Let's start by taking a look at some historical facts. Skin care has a long and intriguing background. Did you know:

- Myrrh has been used for over 3,000 years and was a favorite essence in the ancient Egyptian world for embalming preparations, perfumes, and beauty and health aids. Because of its wonderful preserving properties, it became an important cosmetic ingredient. Myrrh was also included in a facial masque recipe dating back to 15 B.C.
- In early Egyptian time the women used chamomile tea as a hair rinse. This herbal tea would bring out the natural blonde highlights in their hair.
- Two thousand years ago the aloe plant was used to heal and beautify the skin. Fresh aloe juice and gel were massaged into Cleopatra's skin to keep it soft and supple.
- In the fourteenth century Queen Elizabeth of Hungary used rosemary oil for its cosmetic properties. The oil was used in an herbal facial wash and rejuvenating lotion. It helps to heal dry skin and stimulate a dull complexion, and its powerful deodorizing properties helped keep the skin fresh and clean.
- Milk and aloe juice were blended together and used as a face wash by Josephine, wife of Napoleon.
- The yucca plant, found in the deserts of Nevada, Arizona, and California, has cleansing properties that were discovered by the ancient Navajo Indians. The bark of the plant was pounded with a rock; then it was stirred quickly in warm water to create suds. This sudsy water was used to wash the hair, face, and body.

Taking a peek at the skin-care regimes of the past is fun, but how much do you know about the up-to-date facts? Take the following true-false test and find out!

SKIN IQ—21 WAYS TO TEST YOUR SKIN KNOWLEDGE

Here's a quick quiz that will test how much you know about your skin. Circle either true or false for each statement, then check your answers with the correct answers at the end of the test. Good luck and no peeking.

1. Blackheads develop because the skin is dirty. (Chapter Two)

   True False

2. An oily complexion can benefit from an alcohol-free toner. (Chapter Two)

   True False

3. Fragrance in skin-care products can cause irritation in delicate complexions. (Chapter Two)

   True False

4. Oily foods make your skin greasy. (Chapter Two)

   True False

5. Only teenagers and young adults are prone to acne. (Chapter Two)

   True False

6. People with sensitive skin complexions should never use an aggressive facial scrub. (Chapter Two)

   True False

7. Enlarged pores can be permanently made smaller in size by using special skin-care products. (Chapter Two)

   True False

8. Oily skin complexions benefit from extra cleansings during the day. (Chapter Three)

   True False

9. Using a facial scrub will improve an acne condition. (Chapter Three)

   True False

10. The quality of your skin can be influenced by eating a well-balanced diet. (Chapter Four)

    True False

11. Pampering yourself is an expensive ordeal. (Chapter Five)

    True False

12. Baths can have a skin-softening effect on your skin as well as help soothe frazzled nerves. (Chapter Five)

    True False

13. Shaving sensitive skin with a moisturizer underneath the shaving creme can help prevent irritation. (Chapter Seven)

    True False

14. Switching to a richer day moisturizer during the cold winter months can help prevent excessive dryness if you suffer from dry skin year round. (Chapter Eight)

    True False

15. Superficial fine lines can be slightly reduced by using products that contain glycolic acid/AHAs. (Chapter Nine)

    True False

16. The sun will help clear up acne. (Chapter Ten)

    True False

17. If you don't get a sunburn and you tan slowly you won't damage your skin. (Chapter Ten)

    True False

18. It is absolutely necessary to use a sunscreen with an SPF of at least 15 if your skin is being treated with Retin A. (Chapter Ten)

    True False

19. You will be completely protected from the sun if you apply sunscreen with an SPF of 15 once a day. (Chapter Ten)

    True False

20. Professional facials help to deep-cleanse the skin. (Chapter Thirteen)

    True False

21. Visiting a salon or spa can help reduce stress. (Chapter Thirteen)

    True False

Answers: 1. false, 2. true, 3. true, 4. false, 5. false, 6. true, 7. false, 8. true, 9. false, 10. true, 11. false, 12. true, 13. true, 14. true, 15. true, 16. false, 17. false, 18. true, 19. false, 20. true, 21. true

How'd You Do? If you have more than half correct, you know a good deal more about the skin than most people. If you didn't get at least half correct, you're in good company and have a lot to learn. In either case, keep reading. Detailed explanations for each of these statements will be found throughout the book.

ANATOMY OF YOUR SKIN

The anatomy of your skin is complex and intricate. You can compare the structure of your skin to the construction of a car engine. If a part of the engine is missing, worn, or broken, it stops running. The same happens with the skin. If one part of the skin is missing, worn down, or malfunctioning, it will affect the delicate balance of this organ, causing any number of skin problems, disorders, or diseases. Take a look at the following facts about the skin; they will help you understand why skin-care programs and products must be created with the structure of the skin in mind.

- The skin is one of the largest organs of the body. It accounts for approximately 16 percent of total body weight. A 125-pound person has about 19.25 pounds of skin.
- The skin is approximately 0.1mm thick. The skin on the palms and the soles is the thickest (0.8 to 1.4mm). Obviously, nature provides us with an extremely durable skin cover for the bottom of our hands and feet. Indeed, the skin on our hands and feet reflects the lifestyle we lead. Depending on lifestyle, a person can develop a thicker skin in certain places that act as protection. This increased thickness is called callus.
- The skin is divided into three layers: the epidermis, dermis, and subcutaneous tissue layer. All the layers are intimately connected and work as a team. When the skin is healthy, all three layers operate together with great precision.

Don't Judge a Book by Its Cover—the Epidermis

- The outermost part of the skin is called the epidermis. The epidermis is made up of four layers: basal cell layer (where skin cells are born), stratum spinosum, stratum granulosum, and stratum corneum.

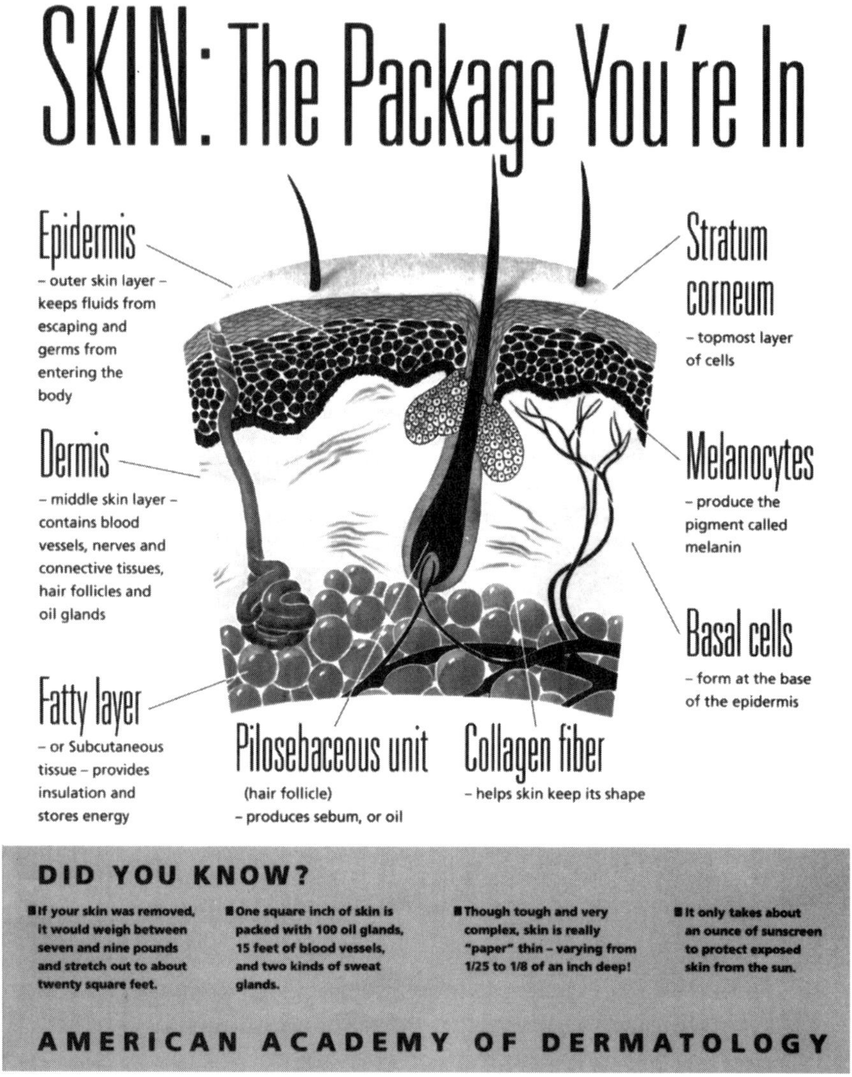

- The outermost part of the epidermis is called stratum corneum. This medical word sounds a bit complex, but it isn't. *Stratum* means layer and *corneum* are flat, dead skin cells. The major part of the stratum corneum—the hair and nails—is made of keratin; this is protein that has a high molecular weight which means they are quite solid.

- The stratum corneum is made up of approximately 40 percent keratin, 40 percent water, and 20 percent lipid.
- The stratum corneum can absorb five to six times its weight in water, but when it becomes dry and the water content falls below 10 percent, the pliability of the skin fails, causing dry, cracked skin.

What Gives Your Skin Its Glow and Vitalty—the Dermis

- The dermis is the second layer of skin, it is located immediately below the epidermis, and is intimately connected. It also is known as true skin. The dermis contains collagen and elastin fibers and sweat and oil glands, as well as a rich blood supply.
- The production of collagen slows down in puberty and levels off in the twenties and thirties. As a person matures there is relatively little collagen production. It is lack of collagen that leads to the thinning of the skin and the wrinkles and sagging of aging skin.
- Collagen also serves as a protective barrier against trauma.

A LITTLE PADDING NEVER HURT ANYONE

- The subcutaneous tissue layer is located below the dermis. This part of the skin also consists of connective tissue and fat cells (up to 3mm thick in the abdomen).
- The subcutaneous tissue layer helps to support the skin. You might even say it acts as a strong foundation. Without it the skin would not have its smooth surface.

The Secret Diary of Your Skin

- When you look at your skin, you're looking at the end result of a 28-day cycle. Skin cells divide continuously as they transverse four layers of the epidermis beginning their journey as part of the basal (reproductive part of the skin) cell layer, up through the stratum spinosim, stratum granulosum, and finally at the stratum corneum (outermost layer).

- When they begin their migration, skin cells are plump, and as they get closer to reaching their final destination at the stratum corneum, they begin to flatten.
- In the dermis, the skin cell membrane releases a water-insoluble fatlike substance called lipids. This substance contributes to the bonding and strength of cells at the end of their 28-day journey when they have reached the outermost part of the epidermis. Think of the lipids and cell membranes as cement or mortar and think of the dead skin cells as bricks. When you reinforce the bricks with cement or mortar you have built a strong structure.

BEHIND THE SCENES—THE INNER WORKINGS OF YOUR SKIN

The skin is an active organ that provides vital metabolic functions that include regulatory processes and protection. Every part of the skin functions in balance with every other part and is a reflection of the overall health of the body. The following information will give you some insight into how the skin works. This knowledge can help you prevent skin problems in the future and understand the ones you have now.

A Protective Barrier

The prime function of the skin is to act as a protective barrier. This barrier provides the body with innate immunity: Most microorganisms that have contact with the skin cannot penetrate the epidermal layer. In addition, the surface secretions of the skin have a slightly acidic pH, which discourages microbial invasion.

The skin is our first line of defense against the outside world. But if we abuse it or care for it incorrectly, problems can occur. For example, you've learned that if you wash your hands too often, they get dry. Now what will happen if you complicate this condition by not applying a hand cream to counteract the dryness and then go out in cold weather? The skin would get extremely chapped and irritated. It could even crack and bleed. Your first line of defense, the skin, is now weakened and can be invaded by bacterial or viral germs.

The skin also helps reduce the penetration of UV radiation. The component of the skin that acts as a UV shield is called melanin—the pigment cells that give your skin color. How much protection you have against UV rays is judged by the color of your skin. The lighter your skin, the less protection you have; the darker your skin, the more protection you have. African Americans have the greatest amount of melanin, which absorbs much of the skin-damaging UV radiation and transforms it into warmth for the body. But if your skin is light, you don't have the same protection, so your skin will take the direct impact of the ultraviolet light. When this happens, your skin incurs an injury called a tan or sunburn. The American Academy of Dermatology recommends that whatever shade of skin you may have you should wear a sunscreen with an SPF of 15 every time you are exposed to sunlight.

Collagen—A Secret Ingredient that Keeps Your Skin Young and Fit

The dermis (also called "true skin") is the part of the skin that provides tone. Seventy percent of the dermis is made up of collagen fibers. The collagen fibers are what gives the dermis strength and toughness. Coarse bundles of collagen are found in the deepest part of the dermis. You can compare the way collagen fibers function to the coils in a mattress. If you didn't have the support coils, what kind of mattress would you have? The mattress without coils would be fragile, flat, and would offer no support. Well, it's the same with the skin. We see this sagging situation occur as we mature because the production of collagen decreases. This is why mature skin looks thinner and extremely fragile.

Elasticity

The elasticity of the skin is due to elastin fibers located in the dermis. They are loosely interwoven in all directions like a network of mesh. You might compare them to interwoven elastic bands; they have the same give and take. The ability to stretch, then resume original size, is due to the memory of the elastic composition. What happens to an old pair of stretch socks or an elastic waistband that has been laundered too much? It loses its stretching memory and doesn't have the ability to spring back to its original shape. As we age, unfortunately the same process occurs with the elastin fibers of the dermis.

The Natural Moisturizer of Your Skin

Oil (sebaceous) glands, which are located next to hair follicles, continually coat our skin with a thin film of oil to help keep the skin supple. These glands are especially abundant on the scalp, face, chest, and back. This is why acne is found in these areas. Acne is a chronic disorder of the sebaceous glands consisting of either noninflammatory or inflammatory type of lesions (pimples).

Keeping Your Skin Cool as a Cucumber

Sweat glands in the skin function automatically as the body's temperature changes. There are approximately 2.5 million sweat ducts on the surface of the skin that are distributed throughout the body, but they are concentrated on the palms, soles, and under the arms and forehead. Perspiration from these glands can occur in response to emotions and spicy foods. Did you ever get wet, clammy hands when you were nervous? Well, those are your sweat glands hard at work. Initially, this sweat is odorless. An odor develops after it comes in contact with the bacteria on the skin.

The production of sweat also helps maintain the hydration of the epidermis and cool the skin through evaporation. The minimum healthy secretion of perspiration per day is 0.5 liter and the maximum is 10 liters. (Men sweat more than women) Even if you do not feel as if you're perspiring you are still losing moisture through the sweat ducts. This is why it's important to drink the recommended eight, 8-ounce glasses of water a day. (Tea and coffee don't count as a fluid because they act as a diuretic.)

How Your Skin Can Give You Strong Bones

The skin plays an important role in the production of vitamin D. The strength and quality of our bones are maintained because vitamin D helps regulate the amount of calcium in our body. Rickets, a disease of the bones that occurs during the developmental years, is caused by a low quantity of calcium due to a deficiency of vitamin D. Our quantity need for vitamin D is extremely small, and there are only two ways to get it: vitamin D is found in food and in sunlight. There is an extremely limited amount of foods that contain vitamin D (Example: vitamin D fortified milk and infant formula, breast milk, fish liver oil, and eel body oils), so our skin's ability to convert ultraviolet rays into vitamin D is an important function of the skin.

SUM IT UP!

There is a great deal to learn about the skin that takes years of study to fully comprehend. This general overview is enough, however, to help you see how the skin is structured and how it functions. This basic knowledge will help you learn how to take care of your skin and understand why neglected skin becomes open to both superficial and serious (sometimes irreversible) damage. Learning skin basics is the first step toward protecting and nurturing your skin.

CHAPTER *Two*

TAKE CONTROL

LEARN HOW TO RECOGNIZE YOUR SKIN TYPE AND CONDITION

Just mention the words "skin imperfections" to most people and you touch a raw nerve. Many of us are unhappy with the way our skin looks. Think about it! Did you ever have a bad skin day? This is equal to or worse than a bad hair day. Have you wondered how you're going to face the world with your blemishes, flakiness, fine lines, or whatever the problem may be? Well, stop worrying and take control. Find out exactly what skin type you have. Decide what you would like to change about your skin. Discover the cause, remedies, and prevention of common skin problems. And let me help you.

I can give you a most powerful skin-care tool: This tool is information. Having all the facts will help you protect, manage, and maintain your complexion. It will put you in control and make taking care of your skin less stressful. Information will also give you the upper hand on a problematic condition and help you regulate the situation. Factual information will show you that many of the skin imperfections you've been suffering with can be managed, maintained, and often controlled with little or no effort.

The questions I'm most frequently asked are: "What kind of skin do I have?" and "Can I change my skin?" These are important questions because without the answers, how can you know how to take care of your skin? One of the most important points to remember when trying to understand your skin type and condition is that your skin is a living organ that reacts to the overall health of your body as well as to your stress level. Although your skin may be predisposed to a condition due to heredity, the condition of your skin can still change on a day-to-day basis and can be host to a potpourri of problems over the years. The good news is that once you recognize and understand the special needs of your skin, there are many different types of skin-care products and over-the-counter medications and prescriptions to help you care for it. And most important of all, there are specific preventive steps you can take to help protect your skin.

THE "FACE-SAVING" SKIN ANALYSIS WORKSHOP

Analyzing your skin may sound complicated, but it's not. The simple plan outlined in this chapter will teach you professional techniques to examine and assess your complexion. It's easy and it works.

How Often Should You Analyze Your Skin?

One skin exam is definitely not enough. Think of this task as an ongoing seasonal ritual. When you examine your skin periodically, you can prevent a simple problem from snowballing into a serious condition. In fact, the skin is known to change with age as well as to slightly change with the seasons. In many cases your skin-care products or prescription skin-care treatments may need to be slightly adjusted.

The Dynamics of Self Skin Examination

I will be using the term "skin type" throughout this book. It is a phrase that is commonly used in the beauty industry to gauge the category or description in which your skin may be classified. How do you know what category your skin falls into? It's simple. Everything is measured around two basic factors: the moisture and oil content of the skin. When your skin has the perfect balance of oil and moisture you have a normal skin type. But if there is either too much or too little oil and moisture it can throw the delicate mechanics of the skin off balance. The skin can become dry or oily. But it doesn't end there, because you can have different degrees of dryness and oiliness depending on the severity of the problem. When an unbalanced skin type is neglected it can make your skin prone to a variety of minor skin conditions. For example, dry skin is prone to flakiness, irritation, and dullness, and oily skin could be prone to blackheads, enlarged pores, and shininess.

FOUR SIMPLE STEPS FOR EXAMINING YOUR SKIN

Before you begin the self-examination of your skin you will need to follow a few guidelines:

1. When you examine your skin it's important to maximize your visibility. Use a mirror that has a triple to quadruple magnification. Don't be shocked when you look into this type of mirror—you'll see *everything.*
2. If you're not sure how to test for oily skin, here's a method that won't fail. Cut out five 3″ × 3″ squares of white or tan parchment paper. Take the paper and blot your forehead, cheeks, chin, and nose. Each area should be blotted with a separate paper square. If your skin has excess oil, it will stain the paper and you can easily see it.

   Note: Never try this test just after you wash your face. The test will not be accurate because you have removed all the surface oils. The best time to test for excess oil is at least three to four hours after you have cleansed your skin. By this time the oils will have returned in full force.
3. How can you test your skin to see if you are dehydrated? Use your thumb and index finger to gently squeeze a small portion of your skin. Look to see if the skin you are gently pinching has a parchmentlike (dry looking) texture. Another no-fail test to determine if you are dehydrated is to exaggerate your facial

movements, such as a smile, a frown, a yawn. If your skin feels uncomfortable and tight, you'll know your skin is dry. Dry skin tends to be less flexible.

4. When you test your skin for elasticity and tone, always test the eye area first. This area tends to show the first signs of aging. When you perform this test use your thumb and index finger to gently pinch a very small amount of skin. Gently lift it; then immediately release it. Test the outer corner of the upper eyelid, then the outer lower eye area and then the jawline. If your skin springs back immediately without any hesitation you're in good shape. But, if your skin doesn't respond immediately and hesitates before returning to it's original state, you have confirmed the loss of elasticity and tone.

THE COMPLEXION-PERFECTING SKIN TEST

This four-step skin test will help you truly understand your skin. After this test you will know if you need to change your cleanser or moisturizer or visit an esthetician, dermatologist, or cosmetic surgeon. You can take this test alone or with your friends, but take your time. You'll use the results of this test as a base for all future skincare decisions.

STEP 1: 18 NO-FAIL WAYS TO IDENTIFY YOUR SKIN TYPE

To identify your skin type, rate how each of the following 18 statements applies to you. Use a scale of 1 (completely untrue) to 6 (describes me perfectly). Enter the rating after each statement.

1. My skin never feels too oily or dry.
2. I never have any blemishes.
3. The texture of my skin looks refined and feels smooth.
4. My skin is shiny.
5. I notice that my pores are large and my skin looks coarse.
6. I have blackheads and clogged pores.

7. My skin feels tight and uncomfortable.
8. My skin looks dull or ashy.
9. I've noticed that my skin is sometimes flaky.
10. If I gently pinch my skin it doesn't bounce back right away, especially on my eyelids.
11. There are fine lines forming around my lips and corners of my eyes.
12. I am developing discolorations and/or brown spots on my face, arms, and hands.
13. I have pimples that are irritated and inflamed most of the time.
14. My skin is becoming scarred after my pimples have healed.
15. My skin is occasionally flaky.
16. My skin is oily only on the forehead, nose, and chin (the T-zone).
17. I've notice that the outer perimeter of my face (cheeks, forehead, temples) feels normal to dry.
18. My pores are large only in my T-zone area, but are small, almost invisible, on the rest of my face.

Skin-Type Rating Sheet

Transfer your ratings for each statement to the appropriate numbered line below. Then circle the skin-type box with a score of 10 or more—this is your true skin type. If you circle more than one box, you have a combination skin type, which is very common, especially the oily/normal, oily/dry, normal/dry, dry/mature, acne/oily, and acne/mature combinations.

Skin Type Ratings

Normal Skin

1. ___
2. ___
3. ___

Total score: ___

Oily Skin

4. ___
5. ___
6. ___

Total score: ___

Dry Skin

7. ___
8. ___
9. ___

Total score: ___

Mature Skin

10. ___
11. ___
12. ___

Total score: ___

Acne Skin

13. ___
14. ___
15. ___

Total score: ___

Combination Skin

16. ___
17. ___
18. ___

Total score: ___

Skin-Type Rating Sheet Example

Take a look at the rating sheet that follows. This individual has an oily skin type because, as you can see, she scored high in that box (above 10). Her oily skin is prone to shininess and is coarse in texture. Enlarged pores always seem to be a problem with this skin type, especially in the T-zone area. The excess oil that flows from the sebaceous gland acts like a catalyst that triggers clogged pores and blackheads.

Example

Skin Type Ratings

Normal Skin
1. 1
2. 3
3. 1

Total Score: 5

Oily Skin
1. 6
2. 6
3. 3

Total Score: 15

Once your have discovered your true skin type, locate the description of this type in the following section and learn how to care for your complexion.

STEP 2: LEARN ABOUT YOUR SKIN TYPE

Below are descriptions of six basic skin types. Find the types you circled in Step 1, match them to the material below, and read the information carefully.

ENHANCE YOUR KNOWLEDGE ABOUT NORMAL SKIN

Flawless! Your skin is perfect. Congratulations on having normal skin because not too many people have this skin type. Your friends are probably envious of your complexion.

Why Is My Skin Normal?

Your skin has the perfect balance of moisture and oil and is free of any diseases and disorders. *Balanced* and *healthy* are two words that describe the state of your skin. It is neither dry nor oily. Did you know that having the perfect balance of oil (sebum) is what actually helps prevent your skin from becoming dehydrated? The skin's natural oils help to slow the evaporation of moisture. The smooth texture of your skin is due to the fact that your pore size is small because of the normal flow of oil. There are also no underlying impurities, blackheads, or buildup of dead skin. Your skin always has a healthy glow.

Do I Really Have to Fuss with My Skin?

Having healthy, normal skin doesn't mean that you can neglect your skin. A good basic skin-care program is all you need.

Will I Always Have Normal Skin?

Remember, the skin is a living organ, and it is always undergoing changes. As you mature, your skin may change. Take into consideration that if you abuse your skin with overexposure to the sun you will definitely alter its normal, healthy state. Sun damage can transform a silky smooth, glowing normal complexion into one that's leathered, dry, and uneven in tone. (That description should make you run for the broad-spectrum sunscreen!)

Selecting the wrong skin-care products can also affect your normal skin in a negative way. Too much oil in a product can clog your pores, and a toner with alcohol or a harsh soap can make your skin dry. Illness can also play a role in changing a normal skin. Remember, your skin is a reflection of your overall health.

LEARN THE #1 REASON YOUR SKIN IS OILY

Shiny and sometimes impure! Having oily skin can be frustrating. You would like your skin to look perfect, but it doesn't quite happen. Many of us have a problem with oily skin during puberty. As we get a little older, the problem seems to lessen, but not for everyone. When we think we're finally rid of this problem, it surfaces again. Hormones, stress, a busy schedule, and the hot summer months will see to that. Are you always on a quest to try products that will get rid of your shiny complexion and make your skin look smoother? Do you feel as if your skin is always changing from one day to another? Read on and you'll soon learn what's causing your skin to look the way it does.

Why Do I Have Oily Skin?

Your genetic make-up is the main culprit. Oily skin is inherited, despite the myth that says eating fried foods causes an oily skin type. The excess oil is caused by inherited, overactive oil (sebaceous) glands, which produce an excessive amount of oil (sebum). You might say your oil glands are out of control This excessive amount of oil causes your skin to become unbalanced, which then makes it susceptible to complications such as blackheads, whiteheads, and impurities under the surface of the skin. Now, let's clear up a misconception: Many people can have "normal" healthy, oily skin without developing acne. An occasional monthly blemish isn't considered acne.

How Does the Excess Oil Reach the Surface of My Skin?

The oil (sebaceous) glands are attached to your follicles. Your skin has millions of these tubelike structures. This is how the sebum (oil) flows from the inner part of your skin to your skin's outer surface. You might say the follicle acts like a pipeline.

How Does My Skin Become Clogged?

Doesn't that term sound terrible? It sounds like a drain that has backed up. But in a way that's what happens. When the sebum (oil) is flowing through the follicle and there is no obstruction everything is fine. But, if skin cells begin to accumulate in the follicle instead of flowing to the surface, trouble is about to begin. When the sebum becomes trapped it begins to build up. This buildup of oil can form blackheads and tiny bumps under the surface. Here, bacteria may form, causing production of white blood cells that help fight infection. This is how a pimple develops.

Why Does the Texture of My Skin Look Coarse?

Your pore size is inherited (thanks Mom and Dad). The excess flow of oil causes a permanent enlargement of the pores because pores are attached to larger, more active oil glands. This can make your skin look coarse and sometimes thick in texture. The size of your pores will never change. But, you can make them appear smaller by keeping them empty of excess oil and free of accumulated dead skin cells. There is a whole collection of products I'll talk about later that will help you achieve a smoother looking surface.

Why Is the Center of My Face More Oily?

The center of your face is called the T-zone. What is this infamous T-zone? We hear this term all the time. It is always used by dermatologists and estheticians, and we see it in skin-care commercials and magazines. Actually, the term T-zone perfectly describes the section of your face that seems always to be shiny, and it happens to be in a configuration of a *T.* This section is located across your forehead, down the entire nose, and on part of the chin. If you're wondering why this part of your face produces so much sebum (oil), it is due to the large concentration of oil (sebaceous) glands located in this area.

SEVEN SURPRISING FACTS ABOUT DRY SKIN

The battle continues as you try to find just the right remedy to relieve your uncomfortable dryness. Your skin acts like a sponge soaking up every bit of moisturizer as you apply it to your face, not leaving a trace on your skin's surface. Your skin seems relentlessly thirsty as you long to have a fresh dewy finish to your complexion.

What Is at the Root of My Dry Skin?

We inherit many of our skin's traits. Dry skin occurs when the skin doesn't produce enough oil (sebum) because its oil glands are underactive. This malfunction leads to a chain reaction. The natural oil of the skin is an extremely important lubricating component because it helps to keep the skin soft and supple. Evaporation of your skin's moisture occurs without the proper amount of sebum (oil). Your skin loses its ability to hold moisture when this occurs.

How Do I Know I Have Dry Skin?

If you have dry skin, your skin feels extremely tight and has a parchmentlike texture. When you make natural facial movements, it feels uncomfortable. Also, no matter how much moisturizer you apply you still have visible flakes on the surface of your skin. Another good indicator is pore size. If your pores are practically invisible, it's likely that your skin is dry.

I'm Only in My Twenties; Why Is My Skin so Dry?

Dryness can also be the result of abnormalities (which may be inherited) in the outermost layer of the skin—the stratum corneum. Your skin's structure has been engineered with a self-repairing and self-renewing system. But when this malfunctions the results are seen as dry skin. The outer layer of the skin cannot hold moisture when there are abnormalities. Moisture escapes, flaking occurs, and patches of dryness will form.

AT WHAT AGE DOES YOUR SKIN BEGIN TO MATURE?

Some cosmetic surgeons jokingly say we begin the aging process as soon as we are born. But most agree that signs of aging begin to surface when we reach 30. It is understandable that you may have concerns about the subtle changes your skin is experiencing.

How Do I Know If the Aging Process Has Begun?

Aging is a slow and natural process. First, your skin will become noticeably dryer. Mature skin has a thinner structure and is more transparent in nature. There may be a problem with uneven skin tone and possibly age spots. Lack of tone becomes noticeable, especially around the eye area. Adult acne may be triggered by the onset of menopause, but it will usually subside afterwards. Fine lines will appear around the corners of the eyes and above and around the mouth. (See Chapter 9, "Timeless Beauty.") Also, keep in mind that the way your skin ages depends a great deal on how much unprotected exposure to the sun you have had. (See Chapter 10, "Tanning.")

Why Is My Dry Skin Getting Dryer as I Get Older?

The natural progression of aging, especially in women, changes the condition of the skin. During and after menopause a significant reduction in the amount of sebum production will take place (due to the decrease of hormones). So if your skin has always been on the dry side, it will become even dryer as the years go by.

TEN VALUABLE FINDINGS THAT WILL EXPAND YOUR KNOWLEDGE ABOUT ACNE

Acne doesn't discriminate. Teenagers as well as adults (especially women during menopause) can suffer with this skin disorder. Although it is difficult to pinpoint the exact cause, heredity is involved because the imbalance of hormones, which is thought to be responsible for sebum production, usually runs in the family.

Acne erupts when the flow of excessive amounts of sebum becomes trapped in your follicles, causing clogged pores. Inflammation and breakouts will soon follow. It is not uncommon for improper skin care to transform a few isolated pimples into a disastrous case of acne.

How Might I Make My Acne Worse?

Do you ever squeeze your pimples? This kind of "bathroom surgery" can severely damage your skin. When you try to annihilate a whitehead by squeezing it, you're actually causing this pimple to rupture under the surface of the skin. This seepage of bacteria, oil secretions, dead skin cells, and fatty acids attacks the skin like toxic waste. The release of these foreign materials alerts the body to engage in an inflammatory chain reaction, which can result in more skin problems such as pustules, cysts, pimples, and possible scarring. The solution is in your hands: Don't use them to squeeze. That's a big no-no!!

END THE CONFUSION ABOUT COMBINATION SKIN

The name "combination skin" suits this type of complexion perfectly because you have two completely different skin types on your face. The most common is the oily and normal-to-dry type. For a better understanding of the term *combination,* let's divide the face into two sections: the center and the outer perimeter.

The Center

The T-zone (center of the face) is usually like an oil slick because of the large quantities of oil glands positioned in this area. Texture of facial skin will vary: The center of your face will have enlarged pores giving a coarse appearance, and the excess oil will make this area more prone to blackheads and isolated blemishes.

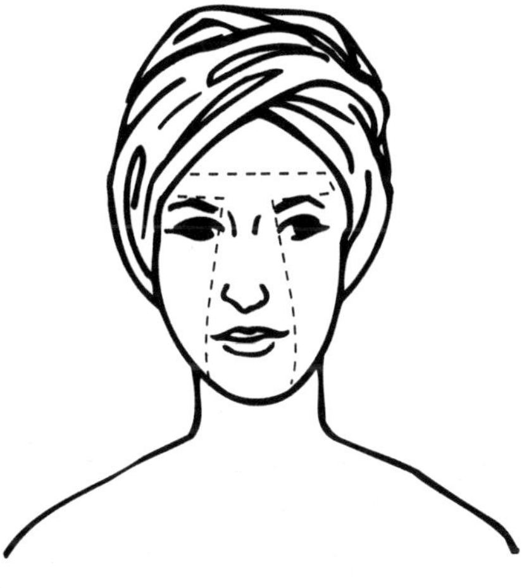

Figure 1 The T-Zone.

The Outer Perimeter

Scaly, rough patches and tightness may be a problem on the outer perimeter of your face if dryness is prevalent. Pore size in this area will be small.

Caring for Combination Skin

If you want detailed information about this skin type, read the descriptions in this chapter for oily, normal, or dry skin, depending on which combination you have. Having this situation can be perplexing when it comes to caring for your skin. The best advice I can give you is just treat each skin type on your face as separate entities.

STEP 3: 15 WAYS TO IDENTIFY YOUR SKIN CONDITION

Let's take a look at the word "condition." It can mean a skin disorder or a chronic disease. I guess the best way to describe the term "skin condition" is to think of it as a complication of your skin type. To identify the condition of your skin, check off the problems you have been experiencing. Then read about these problems and their solutions in Step 4 below.

____ sensitive skin
____ dullness
____ blackheads
____ occasional pimples
____ tiny, spiderlike veins
____ rough, fragile-looking skin
____ uneven tone
____ light/dark spots
____ ashy skin tone
____ dark raised moles
____ small fatty deposits on eyelid

____ loss of skin color

____ keloids

____ inflammation of skin in T-zone (clusters of red pimplelike bumps and swollen nose)

____ stretch marks

STEP 4: LEARN ABOUT SKIN CONDITIONS

The following information describes various skin conditions. If you have any one of these conditions it doesn't mean that it changes your skin type. It means that your skin type may have a few complications that cause either a minor problem or a chronic disorder or disease.

FOUR WAYS TO SAFEGUARD AND SOOTHE YOUR SENSITIVE SKIN

You are familiar with normal, oily, and dry skin types. But what's the buzz word on sensitive skin? Sensitive skin is delicate and can cause you to react in a negative manner to climate, sun, stress, and certain ingredients. Millions of people have sensitive skin, so if you have this condition, you're not alone.

But how do you know if you truly have sensitive skin? Read on and you'll see that I have developed a way to test your skin. All you have to do is answer the questions honestly.

NINE WAYS TO TEST YOUR SKIN FOR SENSITIVITIES

Check off the symptom(s) that apply to your skin. You should be treating your skin gingerly if two or more of these statements describe your skin:

____ My skin is very light to medium tone.

____ I sunburn quite easily.

____ My skin sometimes burns or stings when I use products that contain alcohol.

____ When I cleanse my face with soap my skin feels tight and itchy.

____ My skin becomes irritated, red, and dry with shifts in the weather.

____ Blemishes surface at the first signs of stress.

____ My skin becomes ruddy and flushes without warning.

____ At a drop of a hat, I blush.

____ When I dry my face with a towel, it becomes extremely red.

Solution Special care for sensitive skin—if any two of these statements reflect your skin's appearance you may have sensitive skin. Here's some valuable sensitive-skin advice.

1. Before you purchase a skin-care product, read the label. Products containing alcohol and artificial coloring should not be used.
2. Water temperature should not be too hot or too cold when you bathe or wash your face.
3. Use a smooth sponge or washcloth to cleanse your skin. Any cleansing tool that is too rough will cause you possible irritation.
4. Certain medications can make your skin more susceptible to sensitivities, such as Retin A, Accutane, some antibiotics, sulfur drugs, diuretics, and antidepressants. Many of these medications will make your skin supersensitive to the sun. When that's the case, your pharmacist will apply warning labels advising you to avoid sun exposure.

Skin-care companies have recognized the special needs of sensitive skin and have focused on this problem. The skin care "lingo" used to describe products developed for your skin sensitivities are "less harsh," "mild," and "gentle." To create a milder product, certain ingredients are removed that might cause an irritation.

BRIGHTEN YOUR DULL SKIN IN ONE EASY STEP

A build-up of dead skin cells may be accumulating on the surface of your skin. This condition can make you look pasty and prevent your moisturizer from doing its job.

Solution Exfoliate your skin.

The clarity of your skin will improve when you gently slough away the dead skin. Your skin will become more receptive to your moisturizer.

RX TO ELIMINATE BLACKHEADS

This phenomenon happens when the oil from your skin does not flow completely to the surface of the skin. These natural oils begin to build up and to accumulate in the follicle. Dead skin cells also mix with this oil and become trapped and then solidify into a semi-solid substance. This is how a blackhead begins to develop. It takes approximately eight to nine months before it reaches the surface of the skin and you notice a dark colored dot. The blackhead got its name from its dark color, which occurs because of a combination of melanin (pigment of the skin) and the process of oxidation. Blackheads are commonly found on the face, but they can also develop on the back and chest.

Solution Excessive cleansing won't remove blackheads because they are embedded deep within the skin. There are no products that will dissolve a blackhead. If you have only a few, they must be physically removed by a professional esthetician. If you have a serious ongoing problem with blackheads, it is advisable to visit a dermatologist. A dermatologist has special procedures and implements to remove the blackheads as well as prescribed medications to keep this disorder under control.

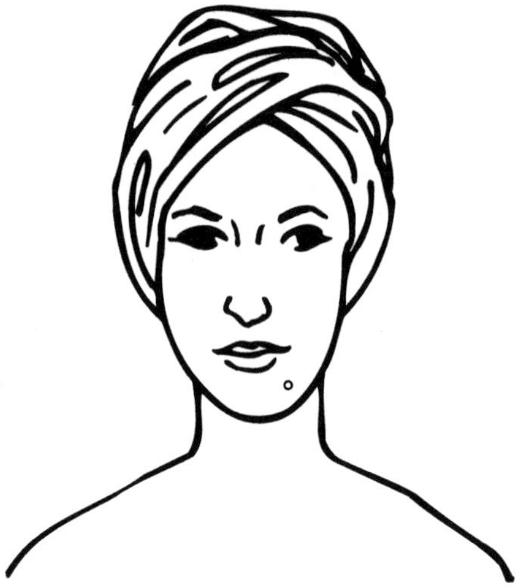

Figure 3
The occasional pimple. Apply pimple medication only to the problem area.

BANISH THE OCCASIONAL PIMPLE

A pimple develops when a clogged pore becomes infected. If you get only an occasional blemish or two then this is considered by most dermatologists to be a Grade One type of acne, which is not serious.

Solution There are many excellent over-the-counter blemish medications you can purchase.

A word of advice: Don't use this product all over your face; it was developed to be used as a localized spot treatment. Too many problems of dryness and flakiness occur when acne remedies are used on the entire face. Apply a little dab directly onto the pimple. Also, if a few pimples escalate into frequent episodes of many pimples, consult a dermatologist.

TWO MEDICAL PROCEDURES THAT CORRECT SPIDERLIKE VEINS

The medical term for this condition is called "telangiectases." This is a vascular skin disorder that is caused by either heredity, topical steroids, aging skin, sun damage, pregnancy, birth control pills, or rosacea.

Solution Dermatologists and cosmetic surgeons have several different methods of collapsing the affected veins; these methods include laser therapy and injection of saline or chemical solution. Another remedy is to cover the problem with foundation or camouflage makeup.

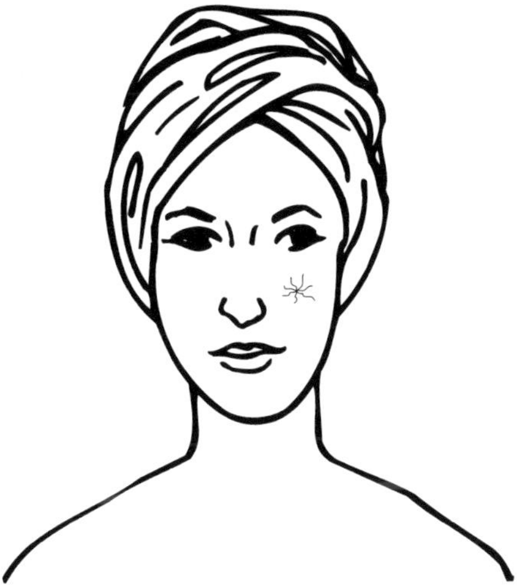

Figure 4 Spider-like veins.

ONE SIMPLE STEP TO KEEP YOUR SKIN YOUNG LOOKING

If your skin is rough, fragile-looking, and has uneven tones, it sounds as if your skin is sun damaged. The traumatizing effects of solar radiation causes the structure of the skin to change.

Solution Completely avoid unprotected exposure to the sun. The medical community of dermatologists and cosmetic surgeons have several skin-improving prescriptions and procedures that help improve sun-damaged skin. You should immediately purchase a sunscreen with an SPF of 15 or more and use it every day. For detailed information on sunscreens refer to the chapters "Tanning" and "Timeless Beauty."

HOW TO PERFECT THE COLOR OF YOUR COMPLEXION

Uneven skin tone can be a sign of sun-damaged or maturing skin. Also, this condition is common during pregnancy (referred to as chloasma) as well in women who are taking birth-control pills. The latter is caused by a fluctuation of hormones in the body and increased sensitivity to the sun. Black skin is prone to this condition due to sun exposure, skin injury, dry skin, or natural variations of shading.

Solution Always wear a sunblock with an SPF of at least 15. This is not just for the beach, but for every day all year long. We get most of our exposure just by walking down the street. There are skin lighteners on the market, but if you're that concerned, it's best to see a dermatologist. For the time being, a foundation close to your natural skin tone will help camouflage the problem if it isn't too severe.

FACE-SAVING TIPS THAT PREVENT LIGHT AND DARK SPOTS

Better known as "age spots," this condition will begin to appear on exposed areas of the skin as we get older. Years of unprotected exposure to the sun is the cause of this problem. The melanin, which are your skin's pigment-producing cells, begin to work overtime: The result is age spots. Age spots are larger than freckles and are irregular in shape. If you're a youthful sun worshiper, you may not see the damage that is happening. But age spots will definitely begin to surface as you age.

Solution Protect your skin with a sunblock that has an SPF of at least 15 or higher. Apply this product every time you expose yourself to the sun. It is never too late to begin. This will help prevent new age spots from developing and will keep your existing age spots from getting worse.

TWO SOLUTIONS TO REPLENISH ASHY-LOOKING SKIN

Dead, scaly skin cells on the surface of a dark or black skin can cause a lightening or ashy cast on the complexion. The dead cells that are about to be shed are lighter than your natural skin tone. The ashy tone is a symptom of a dry skin condition.

Solution Correcting this problem is simple with proper exfoliating and moisturizing products. Your moisturizer should be rich in natural lubricating oils so it will effectively relieve the dryness.

TWO WAYS TO KEEP YOUR SKIN FREE OF MOLES

Moles may take on a light-brown to a brownish-black color. The dark tone comes from melanin, which is the natural pigment of the skin. If your mole suddenly changes in size, color, or shape, if it itches, bleeds, and/or becomes painful, it is vital that you have a dermatologist take a look at it immediately. Sudden changes may be a warning that your mole is not a mole. It may be an early sign of skin cancer. Early diagnosis will increase the percentages of a favorable prognosis.

Solution Moles can be removed by several methods: cryosurgery (freezing), chemical application, and surgical removal are commonly used.

SKIN-SMOOTHING ADVICE FOR TINY BUMPS AROUND YOUR EYES

This condition could be a warning signal that your blood cholesterol is elevated. Yellowish pimplelike bumps are filled with cholesterol deposits and appear most commonly on the eyelids.

Solution Don't squeeze these bumps because you will scar your skin. You should visit your internist to see what is at the root of this symptom. You may need treatment to lower your cholesterol if that is the problem. It's better to be safe than sorry.

There are a few ways these small bumps can be removed: chemical application, cryosurgery (freezing), and a surgical procedure are most commonly used. The results are quite good, but there is a possibility that they will reappear again, especially if the root of the problem isn't corrected or controlled.

LEARN HOW YOU CAN PREVENT AND CORRECT LOSS OF SKIN COLOR

The medical term for this disorder is "vitiligo." It affects 1 percent of the population and is seen in all races, but is most notable in those with dark skin. Vitiligo, which causes a loss of the skin's natural color, usually begins between the ages of 10 and 30. The symptoms are most frequently seen on the hands, wrists, knees, neck, and around the eyes, nose, and mouth. The pattern in which this color loss will occur is unpredictable.

Solution A dermatologist's care is necessary. The use of topical steroids may be used for darker-skinned individuals. Sunscreen is an important preventative treatment because it will protect the skin from further complication. Camouflage makeup can help to even out the skin tone.

DISCOVER THE LATEST MEDICAL TREATMENTS FOR KELOIDS

Keloids are a mysterious side effect that seems to affect many black and Asian women and men as well as a few Caucasians. A simple incision or trauma to the skin can trigger this condition by beginning a scarring episode. The formation of keloids is due to the overproduction of skin cell tissue under the skin's surface. This fibrous growth forms as a side effect of the healing process. How do you know that you are prone to this disorder? You don't know, but doctors say that heredity may be involved.

Solution A somewhat new method of keloid control comes in the form of a bandagelike patch of silicone gel. This gel is applied directly to the problem area. In many cases, keloids begin to shrink, leaving only a tiny, flat-looking scar. This type of treatment is done under the supervision of a dermatologist.

Two Solutions that Control Inflamed T-Zone and Nose Areas

Inflamed, sometimes swollen nose and cheeks could be acne rosacea, which is a chronic inflammation of the blood vessels. The origin is unknown. The symptoms are caused by inflamed and enlarged sebaceous glands and by blood vessels that become dilated. An early symptom is a florid or red look to the skin. Pustules and dilated vessels can be seen on the cheeks, nose, and forehead. Swelling could be prevalent, especially in the nose area.

Solution You must see a dermatologist if you even suspect that you have rosacea. Early management of this disorder could help you prevent permanent scarring. Oral Tetracycline is used in many cases. The Argon Laser could be used to diffuse the enlarged blood (telangiectasia) vessels that cause a red-looking nose, which is a common symptom of acne rosacea.

VALUABLE FACTS ABOUT STRETCH MARKS

Stretch marks look like recessed tiny lines in the skin. This problem is very common, and unfortunately it is irreversible. The best way to describe a stretch mark is to compare it to a tear or run in a stocking. For whatever reason, your skin has expanded beyond its capacity to stretch. Tears occur in the dermis (a lower layer of the skin). This phenomenon can happen during pregnancy and through growth spurts in childhood, body building, and excessive weight loss and weight gain.

Solution There are no known remedies that will completely correct the problem of stretch marks. There is a new laser procedure that will help reduce the prominent color of a stretch mark. Using rich emollients will make the skin feel more comfortable.

WHEN TO SEEK PROFESSIONAL HELP

After an at-home skin examination, you may feel you need professional help. An esthetician can help you analyze your skin, determine your skin type, and care for your skin in a nonmedical capacity. Dermatologists and cosmetic surgeons are trained to diagnose and treat more serious skin problems.

How Do Professional Skin Experts Examine the Skin?

Before an esthetician, dermatologist, or cosmetic surgeon can diagnose a condition and prescribe a treatment or a procedure, they must first know what they are dealing with. Professionals first ask for a complete health history. It is important to list all chronic illnesses, allergies, medications, family health history (many skin disorders are inherited), and any extensive sun exposure. Once this information is taken, the skin examination will begin. Many professionals use the aid of a magnification lens so that the view of your skin's surface can be enlarged. There are some lenses that will magnify the skin up to 11 times its actual size. Touch is also an important part of the examination because it can reveal underlying cysts or tumors. Elasticity and tone can also be determined by touch.

Besides looking for minor conditions, the skin-care professional will look for and document all skin discolorations, birthmarks, distended capillaries, and moles. If a mole doesn't look right, it may be necessary to do a biopsy to check for skin cancer. In many cases skin problems are a red flag for an internal systemic disease. In this case, you may need to see an internist.

At the conclusion of the skin analysis with an esthetician, he or she may prescribe an in-salon facial treatment and a simple home-care program of skin-care products to use on a day-to-day basis. If there is a serious problem, the esthetician will recommend that you see a dermatologist immediately.

See the chart at the end of this chapter. It will help you decide if you want or need professional skin care.

CONQUER YOUR SKIN PROBLEMS

After reading this chapter, you should be well versed in your particular skin type and condition. The thing to do now is to face your complexion head on. It's time to recognize negative habits (incorrect products, unprotected sun exposure, and so forth) and decide to change them. It's time to seek out the correct products, salon/spa treatments, or medical care you need. It's time to conquer your skin.

PERSONAL SKIN CARE MADE EASY

I've created the directory at the end of this chapter to help you correctly select products, salon/spa services, and medical care. The overwhelming amount of health and beauty options that are available to you today can be very confusing, but after reading this chapter, I'm sure you're ready to select thoughtfully based on facts and not on emotions. I don't mention brand names because that is your choice, but I do recommend formulations and generic concepts and categorize them according to what is best for you.

SUM IT UP!

The most important part of any skin-care routine begins with determining your skin type. You will discover the special needs of your skin by learning how to analyze your skin and by participating in the skin test in this chapter. This information helps you understand your complexion, and it will open the doors to the correct skin-care products and preventive care. All the facts in this chapter will help you get the upper hand on problem skin conditions and help you protect, maintain, and manage a healthy complexion.

SKIN SERVICE AND TREATMENT DIRECTORY

Skin Type	Salon/Spa Services	Dermatology	Cosmetic Surgery
Normal	Basic facial with or without steam. Facial massage. Exfoliation with grains. AHA peel.	N/A	N/A
Oily	Deep cleansing facial AHA peel Clay or ocean clay masque Gentle facial massage	Mild to medium glycolic acid peel to help minimize pore size	N/A
Dry	Moisture rich facial With steam or warm compress. Stimulating massage Paraffin masque with essential oils. AHA peels Non-drying masque	Mild glycolic acid peel to remove dead cells to freshen complexion.	N/A

Mature	Emollient-rich facial with or without steam depending on your skin's sensitivity. Gently massage with dry oils or essential oils. Liposome treatment Protein ampoule or capsule	Injectable fillers (collagen, fat transplants, and fibril) to smooth out fine lines. Dermabrasion Mild TCA (trichloroacetic acid) peel to help reduce fine lines.	Upper and lower eyelid surgery Face and neck lift Medium to deep TCA peel (trichloroacetic acid)
Acne	Only grade #1 acne should have facial services (isolated blemishes that aren't causing scars) unless recommended by Dr. Gentle facial without steam (steam will aggravate pimples) Antiseptic essential oil treatment AHA peel	Glycolic acid peels Retin A In extreme cases of acne, Accutane is used. Collagen injections are used to fill in soft linear types of acne scars.	Mild phenol peel to reduce scars. Dermabrasion works well on deeper scarring as well as ice-pick shaped scars

CHAPTER *Three*

THE NO-NONSENSE SKIN-CARE PROGRAM THAT FITS ANY BUSY LIFESTYLE

For centuries women have gone to great lengths to achieve a smoother, more radiant complexion. Each generation has had its own mixtures, beauty rituals, and secrets to pamper the skin. The quest for the perfect complexion has always been an ongoing task of cleansing, toning, refining, purifying, revitalizing, moisturizing, protecting, and nourishing. But today, pampering the skin is a bit more complicated due to our busy lifestyles and the amount of skin-care treatments on the market. Because it's difficult to find the correct products or the time to follow a lengthy skin-care regimen, before you know it the drawers and cabinets fill up with abandoned skin-care products that were tried only once or twice.

The solution to this dilemma is to follow a no-nonsense approach to caring for your skin. This new pampering approach to at-home skin care is guaranteed to fit into any busy lifestyle. Certainly, home care does not eliminate the need or desire to visit a salon, spa, or esthetician for professional advice, nor does it replace the responsibility to see a dermatologist or cosmetic surgeon when faced with a skin problem. Think of home care as a bridge between you and professional services or medical supervision. Visits to your skin-care professional may tally only up to four or five visits a year. So what do you do with your skin the rest of the time? That's right: It's up to you to provide the home care it needs.

BEAUTY FORMULAS FOR FABULOUS SKIN AT ANY AGE

The winning appeal of turning your bathroom into a beauty retreat is becoming quite popular around the country. The way you treat your skin today could help you prevent the fine lines of tomorrow. Many skin conditions and problems can be kept under control or prevented if you spend a few minutes a day caring for your skin. This chapter has two sections: *Basic Rules of Skin Care* and *Pampering Beauty Prescriptions.* The first section spells out the dos and don'ts of cleansing, toning, and moisturizing. And the second section offers you a well diversified menu of the latest time-efficient, head-to-toe, home-beauty treatments. Each treatment has been mapped out in a simple, easy-to-follow, step-by-step format that will help you achieve a more radiant, fabulous complexion at any age. (If you are unsure of your skin type or condition, review Chapter 2 "Take Control!")

BASIC RULES OF SKIN CARE

We will now look at some informative topics that will help you break negative skin-care habits and help prepare you to properly execute many of the fun, pampering beauty treatments explained later in this chapter. Each topic is filled with the dos and don'ts of product categories and methods.

BATHROOM CABINET MAKEOVER

Before we begin our adventure, it is important we talk about a deep, dark secret—the back of the bathroom cabinet. There is always one area that's used as a storage bin for half-used, unopened, or unlabeled products. Either you have been saving all these products for a special occasion, or you're not sure how to use the product, or you bought the wrong product. If you haven't used a product for a year or two, it's time to throw it away. The shelf life may have expired and it could now be rancid. I know it's difficult to part with those precious jars, tubes, and bottles (I confess I hate throwing cosmetics away), but the products you put on your face should be fresh.

C.T.M. SKIN-CARE BASICS

Can't wait until you get into all the fun, pampering facial treatments? Before you plunge into any exotic programs you must first understand the three basic rules of skin care I call C.T.M.: Cleanse, Tone, Moisturize. It doesn't sound exciting? Well, C.T.M. is at the core of every professional skin-care program throughout the world. The following topics, "Guerrilla Warfare Against Dirt," "Toners, What's the Real Truth?" and "Moisture Round-Up" are a comprehensive line-up of detailed information that will give you a clear picture of the rudiments needed for your daily skin-care routine.

GUERRILLA WARFARE AGAINST DIRT

The Deep Cleanse

The essence of even the most sophisticated and high-tech skin-care program begins with something as basic as cleansing. Our preoccupation with cleanliness is all around us, as we battle the ongoing war against dirt, pollution, and grime. Cleansing is one of our most popular grooming rituals: a warm soothing lingering bath at the end of a long day, a quick hot shower to wake us up in the morning, the bedtime face wash-up, and the morning face splash to get us going. Immaculate, scrubbed, spotless, bright, fresh, and sparkling is how we want our faces and bodies to look and feel after cleansing. Unfortunately, our skin's own natural moisture and oil acts as a powerful dirt magnet. Particles from our environment stick to our faces like glue. Our ancestors had to look to the cleansing power of natural essences to achieve this not so small task of skin cleansing. The women of Pompeii used olive oil; the women of the desert gently rubbed sand against their skin; the women in Egypt bathed in sour milk and wine, and women of the islands used pulverized plant fibers. And only a few decades ago, our mothers and grandmothers had it easy. When they wanted to wash up all they had to do was grab a jar of cold cream or a bar of soap and they were set.

But today the dynamics of cleansing have changed dramatically. There are countless shelves of bars, gels, lotions, liquids, and creme cleansers. Which type should I select? Each one is so different. The cleanser concept of today is quite different from that lonely jar of cold cream because our needs have changed. Foundations and makeup are designed for their ability to last all day. Cleansers have been formulated to deep cleanse and remove the makeup without harming the delicate balance of our skin. Also, we are more aware of skin types and conditions and one cleanser for all skin types just doesn't cut it.

Six Cleansing Taboos

Improper cleansing methods and procedures can cause adverse reaction to your skin. (I'm not pointing any fingers but you know who you are!) Here are a few tips that will help you break any bad habits you may have.

If you have oily skin, no cleansing obsessions, please. Overwashing won't remove your blackheads; they are too deeply embedded into your skin. All too often this obsession to remove every last trace of oil can lead to irritation and possible dehydration of the skin. Your oily skin will have double trouble. Twice a day will suffice unless recommended otherwise by your dermatologist.

Excessive rubbing won't remove your pimples. An acne condition will only suffer from this action because you could possibly rupture the pimple(s) under the surface of your skin. When a pimple ruptures it can trigger—guess what—new pimples. Light as a feather should be your philosophy when it comes to cleansing your face. Premoisten your face with water, then create the lather in your hands first, then bring the cleanser to your face. When you follow this method it will be easier to distribute the cleanser onto your face.

Hot, hot water will only scald and boil your delicate skin. And if you have dry skin you can kiss every trace of your skin's precious moisture and oil good-bye. Tepid water is your best bet.

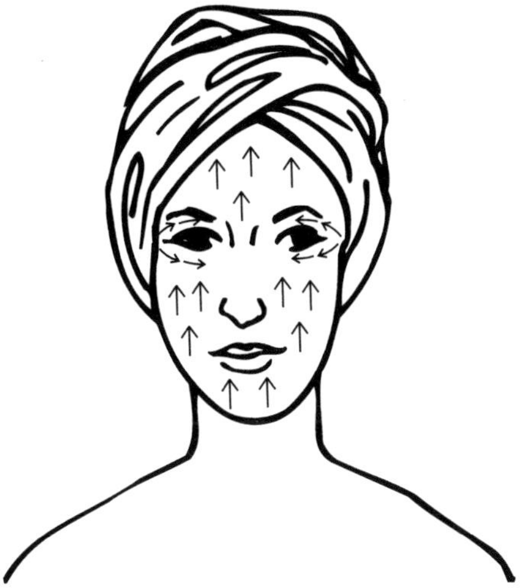

Figure 5 Use an upward motion when cleansing your face, and when approaching the eye area, work in towards the bridge of the nose.

You're not scrubbing pots and pans—that's your face! Vigorous and overzealous scrubbing isn't good for anyone's skin. And if you have mature skin you could be traumatizing it with all that tugging, rubbing, and pulling. If you want to help preserve the firmness of your complexion please treat your skin as if it were a newborn baby. The key word is *gentle.*

Throw away those terry washcloths and rough-textured sponges if you have ruddy, sensitive, or acne skin. Any smooth-surfaced cleansing tool will be your best friend. Frictionless cleansing won't violate the delicacy of your complexion. So if your skin becomes irritated at the drop of a hat use a smooth sponge cloth, cut up a smooth white sheet into squares, or just rinse your face with your hands.

Have you ever noticed a cloudy film on your drinking glasses? That's caused by a buildup of dishwashing detergent due to improper rinsing. Well, the same kind of buildup can happen to your skin if the residue from your cleanser isn't properly rinsed away. In this case it can cause irritation and clogged pores. So don't rush that final rinsing step; it is an important one.

Cleanser Directory

Selecting the wrong cleanser can throw off the delicate balance of your skin. Always read the label and focus on a cleanser for your particular skin type. Normal, oily, and dry skin each need a different type of formulation. Here are a few tips to make your cleanser selection a little easier.

Skin type: oily to normal **Cleanser:** Water-based and sometimes oil-free. Gel cleansers are extremely efficient. They rinse well and leave virtually no residue. Dermatologists like to recommend gel (oil-free) cleansers to their oily-skinned patients for this reason.

Skin type: normal to dry **Cleanser:** Water-based lotion and creme cleansers use milder cleansing agents and also have a higher amount of skin-softening oils than the gel cleansers do. Your skin won't tighten after cleansing. Rinses easily.

Skin type: extremely dry **Cleanser:** Water-based rich creme cleansers have a skin-softening effect on irritated, parched, dry complexions. If just washing your face is an irritating experience, then the rich emollients in this type of cleanser will soothe your extra-dry skin. But, if you use this type of formulation, you must rinse, rinse, and then rinse. Creme cleansers like to linger on the skin. You will need to use a smooth sponge to help you completely remove all the product from your face. And if you were considering using a tissue to remove the cleanser, forget about it. Tissues irritate and dry your skin.

New and Improved Cleansers

The old expression "if it's not broken don't fix it," doesn't pertain to the skin-care industry. Sophisticated tests and high-tech ingredients give cosmetic chemists the tools they need to develop better formulations. The latest ingredient to be added to cleansers are alpha hydroxy acids (see Chapter 9 "Timeless Beauty.") AHAs help loosen, then shed dead skin cells more freely. And as we mature, cell turnover tends to slow down and may need a little assistance in the removal process.

Soap Spotlight

The story about cleansers wouldn't be complete if we didn't mention soaps. Why do soaps get such a bad wrap? As our awareness of the skin and product formulations grows so do our needs. Soaps have been around for a very long time. Many of us grew up with memories of being in a bathtub as a child playing with a bar of soap that floated. There are many people who say it is the best way to clean our skin, and then there are others who dispute the benefits of the soap concept. Soap scum (what a horrible word) is at the center of this controversy. You know what that is: It's the residue that lingers on your sink and bathtub. It is extremely difficult to remove. That residue will also linger on your skin if it is not rinsed well, and it can cause irritation and possibly clog the pores. This tough-as-nails residue is a by-product of a combination of ingredients that are found in soaps: vegetable oils and animal lipids combined with either sodium salts or potassium.

There are alternative measures you can take if you have the "soap concern." Products that boast the benefits of "no residue" are usually soap-free. They contain a gentler, more user-friendly type of cleansing system.

When it comes to the issue of soap, there is no right or wrong point of view. It's simply a matter of personal choice. But, a word of advice—if you do want to use soap always follow these guidelines: Read the packaging and make sure the soap is for your skin type; try to get a soap that is fragrance-free if you have sensitive skin; rinse well (don't leave any soap residue on your skin), and last but not least, if your skin feels extremely tight, dry, and irritated after you have washed your face, stop using the product—it is not compatible with your skin.

Three Valuable Cleansing Tips

- If you have sensitive skin don't use a terry washcloth as a cleansing tool to wash your face. Its texture is too rough. You can use a smooth-textured sponge as an alternative.
- If you have a dull or sallow complexion try using a natural bristle cleansing brush with your cleansing lotion or creme. The

stimulating action of the natural bristles will help to perk up your skin.

- If you wear foundation, cleanse your skin twice. You will need two cleansings to thoroughly remove all your makeup. This extra effort only takes an extra minute or two.

TONERS: WHAT'S THE REAL TRUTH?

Toners are the second step in the cleansing process. They help the cleanser remove dirt, dead skin cells, and cleanser residue. Also, a toner helps prepare the skin to receive the moisturizer.

There is a new generation of astringents, fresheners, and toners, and it is hard to keep track of the action of each product. So always read labels carefully to make sure the product is safe for your skin type. Years ago astringents (developed for an oily skin type) were associated with a high alcohol content and designed to dry up and reduce excess oils. Today most manufacturers have either reduced or completely removed alcohol from the formulations and have replaced it with gentle botanicals that achieve the same results without being harsh on the skin.

Let's talk pore size. Toners do not permanently reduce the size of enlarged pores. But the removal of excess oils and proper deep cleansing can temporarily give your skin a more refined-looking appearance.

What happens to your skin if you are using the wrong toner? Well, two things could happen: An oily skin can become more oily, and a dry skin can become dryer. Let me clarify that. If you have an oily skin condition and you're using a product that is too harsh, you're sending a mixed message to your skin that it's dry and so it sends up more oil. Just what you need—more oil. Now for the dry skin. Again if the product is too harsh (contains alcohol) you will strip your skin of what little moisture and oil it had on the surface. And in the case of dry skin the oil unfortunately is not naturally replenished. The result is that your skin will feel like the Sahara Desert—dry and parched.

Toner Directory

Oily to Normal Skin
Alcohol-free toner

Make sure it contains oil-reducing botanicals

Normal to Dry Skin
Alcohol-free toner

Toner use on dry skin can be counterproductive unless the toner formulation is gentle and is enriched with emollients or natural plant oils.

Sensitive Skin
Avoid artificial fragrance and alcohol toners.

MOISTURE ROUNDUP

Moisture—your skin can't be without it. And next to cleansing, it is one of our most popular beauty steps. We relentlessly blanket our skin with the precious moisture derived from gels, fluids, lotions, and creams. Moisturizing has become a household word, and it is used on every member of the family from babies to grandparents. But what is the exact function of a moisturizer?

Moisturizer Chemistry 101

The roles of moisturizers are significant. They are positioned as a therapeutic treatment based on their low or high lipid (oil) content. The basic purpose of a moisturizer is to heal dry skin resulting from either your occupation (exposure to chemicals or frequent hand washing) or the environment (extremely low temperatures and humidity). If your dry skin is due to the nature of your skin or an internal disorder then the role of a moisturizer changes to that of a comforting treatment because it cannot change the medical disorder.

Reading a lengthy ingredient statement of a moisturizer can be somewhat confusing. Here is an example and explanation of a few ingredients that are commonly used in moisturizing formulas: water, essential fatty acids (unsaturated skin-softening agents such as oleic acid, linoleic acid), humectants (agents such as glycerin and sorbital that help to hold moisture to the skin), and emulsifying agents (that help to hold and bind incompatible ingredients such as water and oil together to form a homogenous mixture).

Keep in mind that what makes one moisturizer more compatible for oily skin and another for dry skin is the amount of lipids (skin-softening fatty substances) and essential fatty acids (unsaturated skin-softening agents) used in the product. Dry skin types need more oil, and oily skin types need little to no oil (oil-free formulas).

Moisturizers that Are More than a Moisturizer

A new breed of moisturizers has evolved out of the chemistry labs and has become extremely popular—skin protectors that contain sunscreens and skin exfoliators that contain alpha hydroxy acid. Using the latest technology, chemists have given a whole new dimension and meaning to the term *moisturize.*

Maximize the Effectiveness of Your Moisturizer

Moistened skin (after you cleanse your face or apply your toner) is most receptive to your moisturizer. The moisturizer spreads easier and it absorbs better.

Flaky skin, a problem even when you use a moisturizer, may signal the need to use a facial scrub or to switch to a moisturizer with AHAs.

Does your moisturizer do a disappearing act on the skin? If your skin still feels tight and dry after you have applied your moisturizer, it is a telltale sign that you need to use a richer type of moisturizer. Visit your skin-care specialist and see if you can get a small sample of a product to test on your skin.

If you have a combination skin type with an oily T-zone, you should divert your moisturizer application to the outer perimeter of your face where it is usually the driest.

Moisturizer Guide

Oily Skin
Water-based and/or oil-free gel, liquids or lotions

Normal Skin
Water-based lotion

Dry Skin
Water-based lotion or creme

Three Moisturizing Tips

- Make the most of your moisturizing step. Purchase one with a sun protection factor of 15. (For information about selecting sunscreens see Chapter 10.) You will prevent many skin problems when you can eliminate overexposure to the sun.
- If you are concerned about the skin in your eye area, use an eye gel, eye creme, or day moisturizer with specializing properties. Gently pat this product around your eye area; begin by working from the outer corner of your eyes, inward. Dab a small amount on your eyelids to refresh tired eyes. When you moisturize the skin around your eyes, your eye makeup will last longer.
- Keep your moisturizer pure. If your moisturizer is packaged in a jar, use a small spatula to remove it. If you scoop the product out with your fingers, you might contaminate the product. You also can transfer your products into a pumplike dispenser; they are easy to use and there is no mess.

YOUR BASIC MORNING/EVENING SKIN-CARE ROUTINE

The Three-Minute Beauty Prescription for All Skin Types

There are many different types of special treatments you can use for the many situations your skin may encounter. But it is important to have a focal point: cleanse, tone, and moisturize your skin. This fundamental part of your skin-care routine is performed on a daily basis in the morning and in the evening. If you're the type of person who doesn't like to fuss with your skin, believe me, after a while this three-minute procedure will take as much effort or thought as it takes to wash your hands. This back-to-basics approach relies on only a few simple steps, making it the perfect solution for anyone who has a busy schedule.

- stretch headband
- cleansing sponge or washcloth (If you have sensitive or acne skin you need a sponge that is very smooth. Anything that is too rough will irritate your skin.)
- cotton pads (small, round, or square)
- cleanser for your skin type
- toner for your skin type
- moisturizer and/or night creme for your skin type
- eye gel or creme (optional)

Step One: Cleanse Pull your hair back with the headband. Splash your face with tepid water and apply your cleanser evenly across the underside of your fingertips. Massage with an upward movement, working in a gentle, yet firm circular movement. Begin at the throat and work your way up to the cheeks, across the T-zone, and finish with the forehead and temples. Splash with cool to tepid water to rinse your face.

Step Two: Tone Apply a small amount of freshener (use an alcohol-free astringent if you have oily or blemished skin) to a cotton pad or ball. Begin at the décolleté (bust line) and gently apply over the neck area and face, using a patting motion. Do not pull or rub the skin.

Alternative: Instead of using a freshener, you can splash your face with plenty of water.

Step Three: Moisturize and Protect While your skin is still moist immediately after applying your freshener, alcohol-free astringent, or water, apply your daytime moisturizer using a gentle patting and smoothing motion. (If you have extra-dry skin, apply a rich night creme in the evening.) Begin at your chin and work your way along the nose to the outer cheeks then up to the temples and forehead. Add a dime-sized amount of product and sweep upward along the décolleté and throat.

There, you're done!

FACIAL MASQUE TREATMENT GUIDE

Why add another skin-care product? Is it really necessary? A facial masque treatment is probably the most misunderstood skin-care product, and it happens to be one of the best kept beauty secrets. It really is a simple step. If you have ten minutes twice a week you can add this treatment to your skin-care program. You will definitely see and feel a difference in your skin.

How Does a Facial Masque Work? This product, also known as a beauty pack or facial pack, is called a masque because when it is applied it covers the entire face, stays on for approximately 10 to 15 minutes, and then is removed. Masques treat only the outermost layer of the skin. This type of product has been formulated with occlusive (gelatinous or filmlike) substances (two examples: koalin, allantoin) that will help hold the product securely to the surface of the skin. This substance in the masque helps to prevent the air from reaching the skin which in turn increases the absorption of the active ingredients into the stratum corneum. An adhesive bandagae is a good example of an occlusive agent. Masques are usually maufactured with high levels of active ingredients that are designed to target a particular need of the skin. Depending on the skin condition, there are masques formulated to either balance excess oil, moisturize, tighten, or stimulate an underactive complexion.

Selecting the Correct Facial Masque

There are many excellent facial masques available, but which one is right for you? The following information will help guide you to the masque that is appropriate for your skin.

For dry skin: If you have dry skin the masque you select should have a creamy or gellike consistency. It should be nondrying, which means it should stay soft and not harden on the skin. The ingredient statement should include natural oils, essential fatty acids, humectants, or essential oils.

For oily skin: If you have oily skin the masque you select should tighten and become hard to the touch after approximately 10 to 15 minutes. The tightening and drying action of this product will help to absorb excess oils, temporarily counteract enlarged pores, and will give more of a refined look to the skin. The ingredients should include clay, oat flour, oatmeal, or talc. This product should be oil-free.

For dull skin: If you have dull skin the masque you select should consist of active ingredients that have a stimulating effect on the skin. The consistency of the masque could be either a cream or gel base. This type of masque sometimes produces a warm sensation to the skin due to the stimulating action.

Eight Facial Masque Tips

- For that special occasion when you want your skin to look extra radiant, give yourself a 15-minute masque treatment. Your complexion will glow, and your makeup will last longer and look more natural.
- If you don't have 10 to 15 minutes to relax once or twice a week while your facial masque is setting, try using this time in a productive way. While your masque is on:

  —do 15 minutes of vacuuming

  —plan your weekly menus and make out your grocery shopping list

—do 15 minutes of dusting
—take a bath
—wash dishes, load your washing machine, or put laundry away
—help your children with homework or iron your clothes for the next day

The list is endless!

THE SECRETS OF SMOOTHER SKIN

Are you unhappy with the texture of your skin? Do you have scaly or rough skin even though you drown your face with plenty of moisturizer? Does your makeup look caked and unnatural? Does your oily skin type look coarse even after you have used a clay masque? Well then, moisturizing and masqueing your skin may not be enough. The truth is, even if you had smooth skin, you probably would want it to be smoother. It is everyone's dream to have skin as smooth as a baby's . . . , well, you know what.

Words like sloughing, buffing, polishing (also known as exfoliating) have been added to our vocabulary in the quest to improve

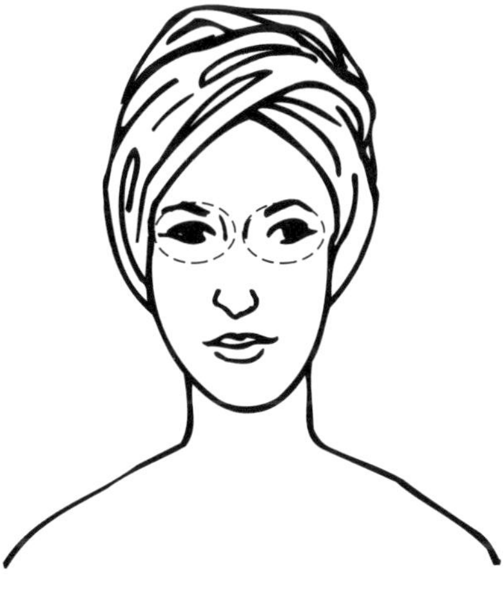

Figure 6 Never apply your facial masque too close to your eye area, especially if you are applying the type of masque that hardens on the skin (Example: clay masque, oatmeal, and so on). These types of masques are not formulated for this area. They could actually cause drying and irritation to the eye area.

our understanding of the texture of our skin. There are scrubs, creams, lotions, and gels that are especially designed to remove the dreaded, unwanted dead skin cell.

How did this campaign and all-out war begin against this minuscule part of our skin? It has been recognized that flaking, scaling, roughness, and dullness can occur when an overabundance of dead skin cells have had a chance to build up on the surface of the skin. Our skin cells shed naturally every day but as we begin to age (after 30) cell turnover begins to slow down.

The good news is that this condition is easily remedied. Women of yesteryear made makeshift treatments to smooth away roughness: volcanic stone, fine coral, extra fine sand, sour milk and wine (the first AHA).

Today there are many skin-smoothing options available, but you should first know about the two completely different methods for removing dead skin cells: friction and chemical. Even though the actions of these two methods are different, they arrive at the same result: smoother skin and a more receptive skin surface for your moisturizer and other treatments. The chemical version (which is very popular today because it offers less irritation than the scrubs) uses active ingredients that soften and dissolve dead skin cells. The skin looks softer and more refined in approximately two weeks. A popular and widely used natural peeling ingredient is alpha hydroxy acid. The friction version of cell removal is achieved by a product category known as facial scrubs. This product has finely ground particles such as almond meal, sea salt, pumice, or bits of loofah incorporated into its cleansing formula. When these small abrasive particles are massaged against the skin it causes a mild friction action. This action gently polishes the skin and whisks away dead skin cell build-up. Your complexion will look smoother, clearer, and brighter after just one treatment. Both these treatments should be part of everyone's beauty regimen.

Do You Have Time to Exfoliate?

If you have approximate two minutes to spare just once or twice a week, you can remove dead skin cells by using the friction method. The chemical version takes only about 30 seconds. It's that simple.

When Is the Best Time to Exfoliate?

The best time to exfoliate is after your skin has been thoroughly cleansed and while your skin is still moist.

Facial Scrub Treatment

Step One: Cleanse your skin thoroughly.

Step Two: Apply a dab of an abrasive facial scrub to the base of your throat, each cheek, and your forehead. (Use fine grains only.) The product works more efficiently if the skin is premoistened. Massage in gentle, yet firm circular movements with your fingertips. Begin massaging at the base of your neck and work your way up to your forehead. Completely avoid your delicate eye area. Then splash your face with cool to tepid water to rinse away the product. You can use toner after rinsing if desired.

Step Three: Finish this treatment by applying a moisturizer to moist skin. (Eye creme/gel is optional.)

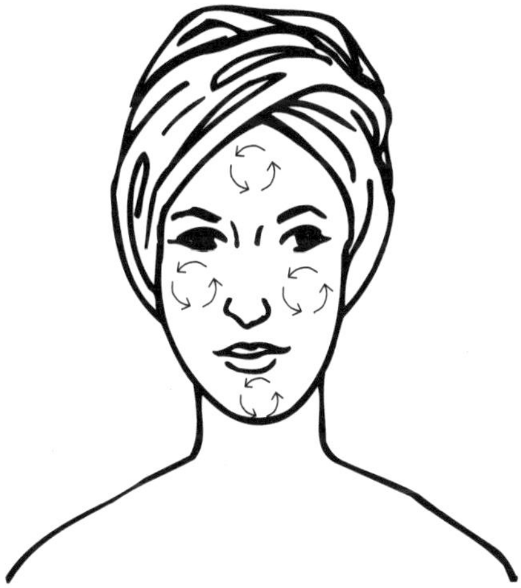

Figure 6 Facial scrubs should always be applied to premoistened skin. With the tips of your fingers use a circular motion with a minimal amount of pressure. Gently massage your face, throat, and décolleté and rinse well with warm water. Always avoid getting too close to your eye area.

How Often Should You Exfoliate?

Sensitive skin: every two weeks
Oily skin: once or twice a week
Normal to dry skin: once a week

Note: If you have acne skin don't use a facial scrub at all.

Six Sloughing, Buffing, and Polishing Tips

- If you have sensitive skin, be kind to yourself by diluting your facial scrub with your cleanser. Mix two parts of your cleanser with one part of your facial scrub. This creates a customized, mild version of a scrub that will be kind to your delicate complexion.
- H_2O is a very important part of the friction method of removing dead skin cells. Water acts as the buffer between your face and your scrub. Without the water there is a greater chance of causing an irritation and fine abrasions.
- Does your skin need a quick pick-me-up because you're feeling tired and your skin looks dull and sallow in color? Sloughing and buffing is a great way to add color to your complexion because it is extremely stimulating.
- To create a special beauty treat for yourself apply a facial masque immediately after you have used your facial scrub. Your skin will be more receptive to the masque treatment.
- Blackheads and clogged pores react favorably to facial scrubs. Gently apply a touch more pressure (as long as there are no pimples) to affected areas when you are massaging the scrub. This will help prepare your skin for blackhead removal performed by a qualified skin-care professional.
- Don't waste a drop of your facial scrub. After you're finished buffing your face, you can buff your hands with the leftovers. It will smooth rough, dry hands. Now don't forget to apply your hand creme!

Skin Facial Caution

- Retin-A and Accutane users beware of facial scrubs. The purpose of your prescribed medication is to accelerate cell turnover and removal. Your skin is in an exceptionally sensitive state, and using a scrub at this time would be counterproductive. If you are considering adding a moisturizer that contains AHAs to your daily beauty routine, please consult with your doctor first.
- Follow your common sense when it comes to abrasive facial scrubs and skin problems. The expression "one person's medicine is another person's poison" holds true with facial scrubs. Severe chronic acne, rosacea, and ruddy and sensitive complexions will suffer from this type of treatment. If you want to join in the quest for smoother skin, ask your skin-care professional about the gentler fruit acids (AHAs).
- No pain, please! Do not use any type of exfoliating product (facial scrubs, alpha hydroxy acids, Retin A, Accutane) before you have a facial waxing. Waxing is an extremely stimulating beauty treatment and it can cause the skin to become quite sensitive. You can exfoliate a couple of days after the waxing as long as there are no residual irritations.

Now you're ready to cleanse, tone, and moisturize. You know why and when you should use a facial scrub and masque. The chart that follows will guide you in selecting the skin products that are best for your skin.

PAMPERING BEAUTY PRESCRIPTIONS THAT WILL MAKE YOU FEEL SPECIAL

This is what you have been waiting for, special beauty treatments that you can do in the privacy of your own home. Each treatment lists purpose, supplies, step-by-step procedures, and special tips with lots of advice so you can maximize your efforts and the results. So sit back, relax, and enjoy. You're one step closer to giving yourself a special treat.

SKIN PRODUCT DIRECTORY

The Basics

Skin Type	Cleanser	Toner	Moisturizer	Night Care
Normal	Lotion Water-based	Alcohol-free	Lotion Water-based	*Creme or lotion Water-based
Oily	Gel Oil-free	Alcohol-free Many toners use herbs to help tighten pore size.	Lotion Oil-free	**N/A** (*use day moisturizer)
Dry	Creme Water-based	Alcohol-free Look for a toner with natural oils added to the formula.	Creme Water-based	Extra-rich creme Water-based (Should look richer than a regular creme.)
Mature	Lotion or creme Water-based Fragrance-free	Alcohol-free Fragrance-free	Lotion or creme Water-based Fragrance-free Contains SPF 15	Creme Water-based Fragrance-free
Acne	Gel or lotion Oil-free Fragrance-free Medicated	Alcohol-free Fragrance-free Medicated	Fluid, gel, or lotion Oil-free Frangrance-free	**N/A** (*use day moisturizer)

Combination: The best way to determine what kind of products you will need is to first determine what skin type (normal, oily or dry) out of the two, covers the largest portion of the face. We call that the predominate skin type. Then go to that skin type in the directory and you will locate the product that is best for you. ***A word of advice:*** This type of skin tends to be more expensive because sometimes it is necessary to purchase several different products to address the problem. To help you economize I have a special application technique that will save you money. Apply either your moisturizer or night creme to the outer part of your face because this area tends to be the driest. Then whatever is left on your finger apply to your T-Zone. The T-Zone is usually on the oily side and needs less moisturizer or night creme.

SKIN PRODUCT DIRECTORY

Specialty Products

Eye Care	**Throat/ Décolleté Care**	**Lip Care**
Creme or lotion	Creme water-based	Vitamin E stick SPF 15
Gel or lotion	Use day moisturizer	Vitamin E stick SPF 15
AHA for eye area	AHA body lotion or creme	AHA for lips Vitamin E stick SPF 15
AHA for eye area	AHA body lotion or creme	AHA for lips Vitamin E stick SPF 15
Gel or lotion	**N/A**	Vitamin E stick SPF 15

SKIN PRODUCT DIRECTORY

Intensive Treatments			
Skin Type	**Specialty Oils**	**Serum (ampoule, capsule, or bottle form)**	**Facial Masques**
Normal	N/A	N/A	Drying or non-drying
Oily	N/A	Intensive fluid concentrate will help to control excess oil.	Drying masque will harden on skin, Clay, oatmeal, sea clay, herbal or seaweed.
Dry	Dry oils, use under moisturizer or for facial massage. Almond, rice, squalane oils are great.	Intensive fluid concentrate will help ease dryness.	Non-drying masque will stay soft on skin. Lotion, creme or gel form. Algae or herbal are great.
Mature	Dry oils Squalane Use under moisturizer.	Intensive fluid concentrate will help skin look smoother.	Non-drying masque will stay soft on the skin. Masques with essential oils help the skin look smoother.
Acne	N/A	Intensive fluid concentrate's antiseptic qualities will help soothe irritated skin.	Either dry or non-drying

Masque Removal Alert! If you are using a drying masque, the type that hardens and gets stiff on the skin, here's a tip for you especially if you have acne. Re-moisten the masque thoroughly before removal. This will ease the removal process so you don't tug and pull at your skin. This would only aggravate your acne skin.

SKIN PRODUCT DIRECTORY

Exfoliators

Facial Scrub	AHA's
Lotion Water-based Fine particles	Lotion Water-based
Lotion Water-based Fine particles	Gel or lotion Water-based
Creme Fine particles	Creme or lotion
Creme Extra fine particles (If your skin is fragile mix a little cleanser with the scrub to dilute it.) If you're using Retin A consult with your doctor before using this product.	Creme or lotion Fragrance-free (If you're using Retin A consult with your doctor before using this product.)
N/A Don't use any scrubs. It will aggravate your condition.	Gel or Lotion Fragrance-free (If you're using Retin A, Accutane or topical antibiotics consult with your doctor before using this product.)

Sensitive Skin Alert! Avoid products that contain fragrance (artificial), alcohol and dyes. Not sure if you have sensitive skin? **Take the sensitive skin test** (page 29).

Supplies

Don't drive yourself crazy! Before you go shopping and spend any money, please refer to Chapter Two so you can analyze your skin type, and check Chart 3A and 3B on pgs. 62-65; they will help you select the appropriate beauty products. Then rummage through all your existing skin-care products and beauty items. (Use only those less than a year old and those completely compatible with your skin type and condition.) If you don't have a product or item that is necessary to proceed with a treatment, check to see if I've recommended an alternative product. Only when you have completely depleted your resources should you go shopping. Prepare a shopping list. I don't want you to buy anything you don't need. When you shop for skin-care products, you should know your skin needs, so become familiar with the type of product formula (oil-free, water-based, creme, lotion, or gel) and consistency that is most compatible with your skin type. When in doubt about a product, locate a skin-care department that offers a complimentary sample so you can test the product before you make a purchase. And don't hesitate to take this opportunity to treat yourself to a professional skin analysis performed by an esthetician.

Portion Control

"Portion control" sounds like a diet, but it's not. This is just a precautionary step that keeps you from overusing your skin-care products or wasting any money. How many times have you poured out too much product into your hands and you didn't want to throw away the excess? Did you ever feel as if you had too much moisturizer on your face and you tried to blot off the excess? Here are a few tips that will help make you more aware so you can conserve your skin-care products. Just follow the suggestions on the chart.

Portion Control Chart

Cleanser. Half dollar or a little larger. It may be necessary to use more cleanser depending on how much makeup you may be wearing.

Toner. Don't make the cotton dripping wet.

Moisturizer. Use a dime-sized portion for oily skin, a nickel-sized portion for dry skin.

Facial Scrub. Use a quarter-sized portion for your face and neck. Use another quarter-sized portion if you want to include the décolleté area.

Masque. Use a half-dollar-sized portion.

Night Creme. Use a nickel-sized portion for dry skin, and a dime-sized portion for normal skin.

Eye Creme. Split a half dime-sized portion between both eyes.

Money Saving Tip

This economical tip is also good for your skin. Always apply your product to skin premoistened with water or alcohol-free toner. Your cremes, lotions, and gels will spread easier so you will use less product. Applying your skin-care products to premoistened skin also eliminates the tugging, rubbing, and pulling syndrome.

SKIN PRECAUTION SPOTLIGHT

Skin pampering is fun, but there's also a serious side. There are precautions you should keep in mind in certain extraordinary situations. Remember the skin has limitations. It's a delicate, living organ.

- If you are using Retin-A, Accutane, or have just had a medical chemical peel, dermabrasion, or any cosmetic surgery, consult your physician before you start any new treatments. You don't want anything you do to complicate your medical care.
- If you have a highly allergic skin type, do a patch test before using any new products. To conduct a patch test, apply prod-

uct to a small area of skin (below the front of your ear lobe or on the side of your neck) and wait 24 hours to observe if the product is compatible with your skin. When in doubt, don't use the product.

- Do not have facial waxing performed if you are using Retin-A or Accutane in those areas. Waxing is an extremely stimulating activity, and when your skin is in the state of accelerated cell turnover (the purpose of these two medications) the wax can lift a patch of superficial skin, causing burning, irritation, or trauma. Tell your esthetician or waxing technician the topical and internal prescriptions you are using. You would be surprised how they can affect the skin.
- Be extremely gentle with your skin and especially around your eye area. Absolutely no rubbing, tugging, or pulling.
- Never use hot water on your skin.
- Don't forget to include your throat and décolleté as part of your facial area. These are probably the two most neglected areas of exposed skin.

Do not use facial scrub anywhere near the eye area. The skin is too thin there to support the friction action of the scrub. To be on the safe side, form an imaginary two-inch boundary around your eyes and don't go anywhere inside that area.

BOTANICAL SKIN TRANQUILIZER— THE FIVE-MINUTE BEAUTY PRESCRIPTION FOR IRRITATED, CHAPPED, OR SUNBURNED SKIN

The sun, cold weather, and low humidity can irritate your skin. Calming, soothing, and comforting relief is what your skin needs. This five-minute skin tranquilizer utilizes the soothing herbs found in nature to help you nurture your complexion back to a more normal, calm state.

When irritated, skin temperature tends to rise due to the inflammation. This is why your skin feels warm to hot and becomes quite uncomfortable. Your goal when treating this condition is to achieve a soothing, cooling, and analgesic effect. The best way to administer a soothing treatment is in compress form.

What Is a Compress and How Does It Work?

A compress is simple and uncomplicated. It is the best way to hold the chilled soothing, analgesic solution in place against irritated skin. A compress can be made from a 12″ x 12″ white, terry washcloth, or a 12″ x 12″ piece of pure cotton. To allow for easy breathing, you can cut out a triangle shape at the center of the compress, or just wrap the cloth or cotton around your entire face, leaving a space in the wrap for your nose.

How to Make a Soothing, Analgesic Solution for the Compress

Nature has provided us with a variety of natural ingredients that have a soothing and calming effect on the skin. The best type of soothing ingredients are found in essential oil form. They are pure, concentrated, economical, and easily mixed with water. Here are a few suggestions when selecting an essential oil for your compress: lavender oil, chamomile oil, rose oil, or neroli oil. All you need is one type. Lavender and chamomile oil should be the easiest to find because they are popular.

How to Mix the Solution for Your Facial Compress

Step One: Prepare a bowl of water with approximately one cup of chilled cold water. Then add 4 to 6 drops of essential oil. Gently stir. It's as simple as that.

Step Two: Place your compress in the bowl or soothing solution until it is saturated. Then wring out the excess. Lie down and apply the saturated compress to your face. Leave on for five minutes. If you have more time to spare, saturate the compress in the soothing solution again and reapply to your face for another five minutes.

Beauty Alert!

Did you ever experience a stressful day? Well, here is something to soothe your frazzled nerves. Mix 1/4 ounce of water with 3 drops of either lavender or rose oil. Then pour this soothing solution into a small purse-size atomizer. Place in your briefcase or pocketbook. During the day you can mist your face and pulse points with this delightfully fragrant and soothing mixture. You can also mist your hot, tired feet right through your stockings. It works every time.

SKIN-BALANCING AND PURIFYING TREATMENT FOR OILY SKIN—THE 30-MINUTE BI-WEEKLY BEAUTY PRESCRIPTION

Oily skin needs to become balanced. Gentle yet effective treatment products will delicately control the excess oil without stripping the skin of precious moisture. Reduce excess shine, smooth texture, and temporarily reduce enlarged pores with this balancing and purifying beauty ritual for oily skin. Tap into the benefits of oil-free treatments and the degreasing relief achieved with purifying clay therapy. Your skin will feel refreshed and smoother after just one treatment.

Supplies

- stretch headband
- textured sponge
- cleanser
- facial scrub
- alcohol-free astringent (optional)
- oil-free moisture lotion
- intensive serum concentrate (optional) and clay masque

Step One: Oil-Free Cleansing Pull your hair back with the stretch headband. Premoisten your face with water. Cleanse skin with an oil-free gel or lotion. Once you have applied the cleanser let it set on your face for 30 seconds. This extra time gives the cleanser a better chance to break down the makeup and excess oils. Remove cleanser with textured sponge, then rinse well with tepid water.

Step Two: Removing Dead Skin Cells Premoisten your skin, then apply a dab of facial scrub to the base of your throat, each cheek, and forehead. Massage in a gentle, yet firm circular motion; start at the base of the neck and work your way up to the forehead. Avoid your eye area. Then remove scrub by splashing your face with cool to tepid water.

Step Three: Degreasing Excess Oil (optional) If you want to treat your skin to an extra step before your masque treatment try applying an intensive serum concentrate especially developed for oily skin. It comes in bottle, ampule, or capsule form. You could also add two drops of lemon or rosemary essential oil to a portion of your daytime moisturizer. Apply either one of these two remedies to your skin and gently massage the skin in a circular motion for one to two minutes.

Step Four: Intensive Masque Treatment While your skin is still moist, apply a clay (drying) masque to your entire throat and face, avoiding the eye area. (This will harden on the face.) Once the masque is completely applied, take a small portion of masque on your fingertips and massage over the previous masque application. This extra application of masque will ensure complete coverage and adherence to your skin to maximize its results. Leave masque on for 10 to 15 minutes (make sure the masque is completely stiff before removal).

Special removal technique: Never begin to remove masque while it is stiff. This will cause you to tug, rub, and pull at your skin unnecessarily and possibly cause irritation. Always rewet the clay masque by moistening it with a wet sponge or wet washcloth. When the masque is completely soft, gently rinse with warm water.

Step Five: Tone Take a piece of cotton and saturate it with a bit of alcohol-free toner and gently sweep your entire face.

Alternative method: Splash your face with tepid water.

Step Six: Oil-Free Moisturizing When you have oily skin there is a special way to apply your moisturizer. This application technique will help you prevent the overuse of your moisturizer.

Apply an oil-free moisture gel or lotion to the outer perimeter of your face (this area tends not to be as oily as the center of the face). Gently massage the gel or lotion into the skin working your way toward the center of the face. If you have any moisturizer left on your fingertips apply it to the T-zone. (The reason you don't apply the moisturizer directly to this area is because the center of the face has the greatest concentration of oil glands.) Finish your facial by applying an eye gel or lotion to your eye area. (Alternative method: You can use your day moisturizer.) Gently apply this product with a patting motion beginning with the outer part of the eye area and working your way in toward the bridge of your nose.

FIVE TIPS FOR CONTROLLING EXCESS OIL

- Cleansers should be water-based and oil-free.
- Use alcohol-free astringents. There are many natural plant extracts that have oil-controlling properties (Examples: Rosemary, Yarrow, Licorice, etc.). Read the ingredients label before you purchase an astringent.
- Gentle exfoliating products are an excellent way to prepare your skin before a clay masque treatment. It will make your skin more receptive to the masque treatment because it removes the unwanted dead skin cells that act as a barrier. Your skin will look and feel much smoother and more refined.
- Clay masques temporarily reduce enlarged pores, giving your skin a smoother, more refined texture. The clay in the masque will also help to remove excess oils.
- Protect your skin with an oil-free moisturizer. Yes, even oily skin can lack moisture. You can purchase an oil-free moisture fluid product that is light to the touch. You won't even know you have it on.

Five Never-Ever-Ever Tips for Oily Skin

- Don't overwash your face with harsh cleansers and soaps. Your skin will suffer for it. In many cases you will aggravate the skin, causing it to produce more oil.

- Don't wipe your face with alcohol. You're only stripping your skin of precious moisture.
- Don't exfoliate every day. Overdoing this treatment can cause irritation, extreme dryness, and flakiness.
- Don't abuse over-the-counter acne medication. If you get an occasional blemish or two, apply a dab of blemish medication on just the blemish. Don't apply it all over your face. There are many excellent acne remedies sold today, but if you overdo it your skin may become extremely dry.
- Don't perform "bathroom surgery" on yourself. Squeezing blemishes, blackheads and pimples improperly will only cause more of an infection, plus you will scar your skin. If you have a few blemishes, see a professional esthetician. If the problem is more severe see a dermatologist.

INTENSIVE H_2O AND THERAPEUTIC OIL TREATMENT FOR DRY SKIN—THE 30-MINUTE BI-WEEKLY BEAUTY PRESCRIPTION

Dry skin can be very uncomfortable. Sometimes your skin feels as if it is two sizes too small for your face, and it can become itchy and irritated. The good news is that dry skin is simple to control. What your skin needs is a good drenching in therapeutic natural oils and specialized essential emollients. Let your parched skin drink up this moisture-rich facial.

Why Is a Special Treatment Needed for Dry Skin?

Did you ever apply your moisturizer, but your skin still felt and looked dry? When you apply your moisturizer does it disappear without a trace? Your skin is trying to tell you something. It is possible that your moisturizer is not rich enough. Sometimes it is not enough to use just a moisturizer. If your skin is extremely dry you may need a special product to seal in the moisturizer as well as to replenish your skin's depleted supply of natural oil. There are several excellent products that will protect your skin in this way. They are pure and natural plant and nut oils. Dry oils are a special classification of exceptionally lightweight oils that seem to disappear on the skin. A few of the most popular dry oils are squalane oil, jojoba oil, sweet almond, and macadamia nut oil. All you need are a couple of precious drops of lightweight oils to help you replenish and protect your skin.

Supplies

- stretch headband
- smooth cleansing sponge
- cotton hand towel (approximately 15″ x 24″)
- small kitchen bowl (approximately 1/4 ounce)
- small kitchen bowl (approximately 12 ounces)
- rich cleansing cream
- alcohol-free toner
- facial scrub
- dry oils (either squalane, almond, or macadamia nut oil)
- night creme
- nondrying masque (can be herbal-based or seaweed formula)
- water-based day moisturizer

Step One: Emollient-Rich Cleansing Pull your hair back in the headband. Apply the rich, water-based cleanser to premoistened skin. Remove cleanser with a moistened, smooth sponge; then rinse completely with tepid water.

Step Two: Remove Dead Skin Cells Mix a few drops of dry oil (either squalane, jojoba, almond, or macadamia nut oil) into a portion of your favorite facial scrub. Then apply the mixture to premoistened skin. Gently massage, beginning at your décolleté and working your way up to the forehead. (Don't forget to exfoliate your lips.) Rinse completely with tepid water.

Step Three: Reconditioning Warm Oil Treatment Combine a few drops of dry oil with a portion of your night creme. Then warm. (Either hold it in your hands to heat or put the creme in a glass bowl and then place that bowl into a bowl of hot water and let it stand for a minute until the oil is a comfortable temperature.) Then gently massage your entire décolleté, throat, and face for at least two to three minutes. Use gentle, gliding, circular motions. Absolutely no tugging, rubbing, or pulling. Keep your skin moist while you massage by adding more creme as you need it. Do not remove massage creme.

Step Four: Intensive Masque Treatment Apply a nondrying masque over the creme and oil. (This masque stays soft on the skin.) Completely cover your entire décolleté, throat, and face. Avoid your eye area. Once the masque is completely applied, place a small portion of masque on your fingertips and massage over previous masque application. This extra application of masque will ensure complete coverage and adherence to your skin to maximize its results. Leave the masque on for 10 to 15 minutes.

Special masque technique: After the application of the masque is complete, apply a warm towel compress over your entire face. Moisten a 15″ x 24″ hand towel with warm water and wring out excess moisture. Lie down and wrap the towel around your face, leaving a space for your nose. Leave the compress on while the masque is setting, approximately 10 to 15 minutes. Remove the compress and rinse the masque off your skin by splashing your face with cool water.

Step Five: Alcohol-Free Toner Gently sweep your face with a piece of cotton saturated with an alcohol-free toner or splash your face with plenty of tepid water.

Step Six: Emollient-Rich Moisture Lotion or Creme Apply a dab of water-based moisture lotion or creme to your décolleté, throat, chin, cheeks, lips, and forehead. Gently massage into your skin. To seal in moisture and create a protective barrier, apply a few drops of a natural plant oil (such as squalane oil, almond oil, or jojoba oil) over your moisturized skin.

Four Tips to Conserve Dry Skin's Most Precious Commodity: Moisture and Natural Oils

- Cleansers, soaps, and toners that are too harsh can strip your skin of moisture. Look for cleansers or soaps that are rich in natural plant oils and essential fatty acids. (If you use soap, make sure you rinse well or your skin will feel tight and dry.) All your products must be alcohol-free. Your skin should feel comfortable after you have cleansed your face. If your skin feels tight and dry after washing your face that is a telltale sign that the product you're using isn't appropriate for your skin. Try a richer type of cleanser.

- Preserve moisture during the harsh winter. The low temperature and low humidity can rob your skin of moisture, causing irritation. Try cleansing your skin only in the evening to remove your makeup. Then tone and apply a rich night creme. In the morning when you awaken, just refresh your complexion with toner (completely eliminate the cleansing step). Then apply a rich day creme.
- Use a liquid or creme foundation. Don't use a powder or matte foundation. These two types of foundation have talc incorporated into the formula. This will rob your skin of its natural oils. Both matte and powder foundations are excellent products, but they were developed for individuals with oily skin.
- Hot water can irritate and cause additional dryness. Use a tepid water temperature to wash your face.

Beauty Alert!

Does your skin sometimes still feel dry after you have applied your moisturizer? The solution: Try applying a second application of moisturizer on the days you feel extra dry. Wait two minutes between applications.

SWEET ALMOND LIP SMOOTHER— THE THREE-MINUTE BEAUTY PRESCRIPTION FOR DRY, CHAPPED LIPS

When your lips become dry, cracked, and chapped they are uncomfortable. This condition, commonly known as chapped lips, is often a chronic problem in cold weather and sometimes accompanies a bout of a cold or flu. The skin on the lips becomes so dehydrated (lacking moisture) that it begins to crack, split, and sometimes bleed when you smile. If you have this problem it is easily remedied. All you need is a minute or two daily.

Supplies

- cleanser
- facial scrub
- antibiotic ointment
- sweet almond oil (alternative products: Vitamin E stick, jojoba oil, or your day moisturizer)

Step One: Remove Dead Skin Cells If your lips are peeling, you must remove the unwanted dead, flaky skin. First, remove lipstick with cleanser. Apply a small amount of facial scrub to your lips and massage for 30 seconds. Rinse well with cool water. (*Caution:* If your lips are split, eliminate this step.)

Step Two: Recondition Your Skin If irritation exists, apply a small amount of an over-the-counter antibiotic ointment. Massage the ointment into the skin. Then apply a sweet almond oil to your lips. (You can also use a Vitamin E stick or jojoba oil.) If you do not have any of these natural oils, use your face moisturizer. Once this condition is under control (which may take a week or so depending on the individual and how severe the condition is) you can follow this treatment once or twice a week. When your lips are completely healed, eliminate the antibiotic ointment.

Beauty Alert!

- Therapeutic Vitamin E stick should be kept in your purse at all times. Apply it liberally throughout the day; you can even apply it over your lipstick. This little step will help you prevent the problem of dry, chapped lips from occurring.
- When you have a cold, does your nose get red and irritated? Well, this lip-smoothing treatment works on red, irritated noses also. It will give you soothing relief quickly.

- If you are experiencing lip irritation and the skin on and around your lips is splitting, an over-the-counter antibiotic ointment will help the skin heal and prevent an infection from occurring. This product is inexpensive and can be purchased in your local pharmacy.

HERBAL EYE RENEWAL—THE 10-MINUTE BEAUTY PRESCRIPTION FOR TIRED EYES

Do you occasionally experience tired, stressed-out eyes? Did you have a late night? Work all day at the computer? Or, are your eyes affected by pollution or allergies? Unfortunately, all of these can make eyes feel tired and strained.

Soothing Relief for Tired Eyes

The truth is, there is no special creme that will reduce puffiness around the eyes. But there is a remedy to counteract stressed-out eyes—the cool eye compress. The cool temperature of the compress pressed against the eye area will help to soothe and refresh overworked eyes.

Supplies

- cotton eye pads or cotton washcloth
- small kitchen bowl (approximately 8 ounces)
- chamomile essential oil (alternative product: alcohol- and fragrance-free toner)
- chilled water
- eye-care product: gel, lotion, or creme (If you don't have an eye product you can use your daily moisturizer as long as it is not a medicated type for acne.)

Step One: Making a Compress Eye compresses can be made out of medical cotton or cotton pads (approximately two inches in diameter), which can be found at your local pharmacy. If you don't

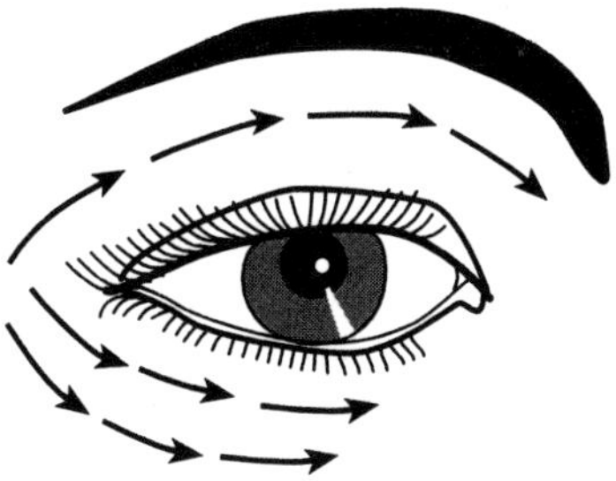

Figure 8 The skin around your eyes is delicate. Use a patting motion when applying your chosen skin-care product and work in toward the bridge of the nose. Never tug or pull at this area.

want to use cotton, you can use a small 12″ x 12″ terry washcloth. If you use a washcloth as a compress fold it in half.

Step Two: Preparing the Soothing Treatment The compress can be made with a chilled solution of either a chamomile essential oil solution (two or three drops in six ounces of water), alcohol- and fragrance-free freshener for sensitive skin, or mineral water. Fill a small bowl with approximately one cup of compress solution, then place in the refrigerator to chill.

Step Three: Conditioning the Skin Apply either an eye-care product or day moisturizer to your eye area. Be extremely gentle in your application. Apply with a patting motion using your fingertips, working your way inward toward the bridge of your nose. Don't forget to put moisture creme over your eyebrows.

Step Four: Applying the Compress Place the cotton pad compresses or folded terry washcloth compress in the chilled solution. Wring out the excess liquid and while in a reclining position apply directly to the eye area. When the eye compresses become warm, resaturate them in the solution and reapply. Repeat this procedure for 10 minutes or longer if you have the time.

Time-Saving Tip If you don't have time to prepare homemade eye compresses, you can purchase a compress that is reusable.

This eye compress can be found in most department stores and pharmacies and is not too expensive. This product is made of smooth, durable vinyl and is prefilled with a cryogenic blue gel. You can keep this eye masque in the refrigerator or freezer. It's ready to use the instant you need it. No fuss and no muss! It's also great to use if you have a headache. Please note that this eye masque can also be heated if you need a warm compress.

Beauty Alert!

Are you planning a special night out after a full day at the office? For a quick pick-me-up give yourself a 10-minute eye renewal treatment before you go out. Just apply a chilled eye compress for 10 minutes and your stressed, overworked, tired eyes will feel refreshed.

Do you want to make your eye renewal treatment extra special and mentally soothing? Light a scented candle, turn down the lights, and play soft, relaxing music.

CITRUS SURPRISE HAND SOAK—THE FIVE-MINUTE BEAUTY PRESCRIPTION FOR ROUGH, ABUSED HANDS

Tough day at the office? Do your hands feel abused? Here's a little treatment you'll want to repeat often. The cleansing action and the fresh scent of the citrus essences will make your hands feel and look renewed.

Supplies

- small kitchen bowl: stainless steel or plastic (approximately 1 quart)
- pumice stone and pumice stick (you can find these items in most pharmacies and beauty-supply stores)
- hand towel
- natural- or nylon-bristle nail brush (salons, department stores, bath shops, and pharmacies carry this item)

- your favorite shampoo (as long as it is not medicated for dandruff)
- facial scrub
- lemon, grapefruit, tangerine essential oils (You can purchase a premixed blend of these oils or purchase them individually. If you can't locate these particular oils the alternative product would be any citrus blend of essential oil.)

Step One: Preparing the Soak Place a capful of shampoo into a bowl. Fill bowl with warm water. While the water is running, add a few drops of your citrus essential oils.

Step Two: Dead Skin Cell Removal Apply a nickel-sized portion of facial scrub to your premoistened hands and gently massage for about 60 seconds. Concentrate on the areas that have calluses. Rinse well. Then place both hands in prepared bowl and soak for two minutes. Gently scrub with nail brush under nails and all over both hands.

Step Three: Reconditioning and Buffing Apply squalane oil or thick hand/body creme all over hands (make sure your cuticles and nails are covered). Continue to soak for another minute. Using your pumice stone, gently buff any calluses you may have on your hands. Then take your pumice stick and push back your cuticles. Continue to soak for another five minutes. Remove hands from bowl and pat dry.

Step Four: Protecting Finish up this special treatment by adding two drops of the citrus essential oil blend to a portion of your hand/body creme. Massage product into both hands.

PEPPERMINT ZINGER FOOT BATH— THE 20-MINUTE BEAUTY PRESCRIPTION FOR TIRED, SORE FEET

The cool, mentholated sensation of peppermint and the sweet aroma of orange blossom will help make your hot, burning feet feel as if you're wading in a mountain brook.

Supplies

- large pedicure basin (If you don't have one, now's a good time to buy one or borrow one from a friend.)
- two large bath towels (One towel is to be placed under the pedicure basin and the other is to be placed on your lap to protect your clothes and to dry your feet.)
- pumice stone and pumice stick
- natural bristle 10″ body brush or abrasive mitt (Both can be found in many salons, department stores, and bath shops.)

  Alternative: If you can't find these items, use your nail brush. It doesn't produce the same sensation, but you can improvise.
- your shampoo (as long as it is not for dandruff)
- peppermint essential oil
- orange essential oil
- rich body/foot creme

Step One: Preparation of Foot Bath Place a capful of your shampoo into an empty pedicure basin. Fill basin with warm-to-hot water. While water is running add three drops each of peppermint and orange essential oils.

Step Two: Invigorate—Condition—Soak Submerge both feet into foot bath. Take a natural-bristle body brush or abrasive mitt and vigorously massage both feet. Concentrate on those calluses. Then apply a thick application of body or foot creme. Soak for five minutes.

Step Three: Buffing and Soaking Remove one foot and buff your callused areas with the pumice stone. Return the foot to the water. Repeat the same procedure on the other foot. Continue to soak both feet for another 10 minutes. This is a perfect time to read a book, listen to music, watch your favorite TV program, or sip a soothing cup of herbal tea.

Step Four: Protecting Remove your feet from the foot bath and pat dry with the large towel. Then add a few drops of peppermint oil to a portion of your body/foot creme. Massage the fragrant product into both feet. Now put on a comfy pair of slippers.

SUM IT UP!

You are the most important caretaker of your skin because you are the one responsible for the day-to-day maintenance that will ultimately affect your skin for the rest of your life. It is not a waste of time or frivolous to address the needs of your skin because you are maintaining the integrity of the largest organ of your body. This chapter has offered you step-by-step beauty formulas, product directories, a skin precaution listing, and the dos and don'ts for caring for your particular skin type. Taking the first step is always the hardest, but now that you understand the particular needs of your skin and the importance of skin-care basics (cleansing, exfoliating, and moisturizing) you can follow a simple daily and weekly regimen that will start you on your way toward a healthier-looking complexion.

CHAPTER *Four*

FEEDING YOUR SKIN FROM WITHIN

Have you ever heard the expression, "You are what you eat"? It's true—every bit of food, water, alcohol, drugs, and smoke that we consume affects every fiber of our being. Years of poor eating habits can take their toll on both our metabolism and ultimately our skin. How can eating affect our skin? The skin is the largest organ of the body, and it reflects our overall health—when there is an internal problem the red flag goes up on the skin. For example, if you have a cardiovascular problem with blocked arteries that restricts the flow of blood through your body, your skin will take on a dull, almost gray cast. If you are a diabetic, your skin may have a problem healing itself; a cut or a scratch on the foot or toe could become life threatening without professional treatment. Think about what happens to a plant that is not watered or fed on a regular basis. The plant's beauty vanishes as the leaves wither and become dry and shriveled. Your skin works the same way. All living things need proper nourishment in order to flourish and bloom.

Well-balanced eating habits offer great dividends in the long run because they can become our most effective skin beautifier and health tonic. The rewards are great and the effort need not be time consuming. This chapter will provide you with a full spectrum of straight-to-the-point nutritional advice and plenty of delicious, low-calorie and low-fat spa recipes that will have a positive impact on your complexion and the way you feel.

A LOOK BACK AT FOODS

Our ancestors ate unprocessed foods such as fresh-picked nuts, fruits, berries, grains, wild herbs, vegetables, and fresh fish and wild game. The choice of what to eat was simple because they ate whatever was in season. They drank plenty of fresh water and teas made from steeping bark, blossoms, berries, or wild herbs. These hearty individuals harvested their nourishment from the wilderness and saved the plentiful produce and meats for the lean months. Unprocessed was the key word because the foods our ancestors ate were consumed with all the nutrients intact and with plenty of insoluble fiber found naturally in the fresh fruit and grains they ate.

A change in eating habits occurred around the beginning of this century. Food manufacturers took foods from their natural state and refined them, creating what we today call processed foods. A most dramatic change occurred in the type of bread that was consumed during this time period. It was thought that natural-looking bread was uncivilized because of its coarse texture and uneven color. (This texture and color was caused by a fiber known as bran, which is the hull of the grain.) New technology enabled manufacturers to process and pulverize the grain and discard its most valuable component, the fibrous hull. The end product was a smooth-textured, white refined flour—without any fiber. This new type of flour affected the way the people of this century were destined to eat for many years. Any recipe that uses flour—such as breads, crackers, breadsticks, muffins, cookies, cakes, waffles, pancakes, and pie crusts—was not to have the same nutritional value or digestive and intestinal benefits for most of the remaining century. The fiber component that helped to keep the intestines clean and functioning properly since the beginning of the human race was missing. The consumption of fiber wouldn't become popular again for many decades.

The industrial revolution pushed civilization into a fast-forward mode where words like quick, easy, and convenient became synonymous with new trends in eating. Packaged cake, cookies, pancake and pudding mixes, refined white bread, canned soups, canned vegetables, canned fruit, and the ever popular frozen TV dinners infiltrated the new supermarkets. The age-old job of preparing food for the table was eliminated—along with valuable nutrients and fiber. This trend remained strong right though to the seventies and early eighties.

Although "foods for convenience" will probably always have a strong foothold in food manufacturing and consumption, trends come and go. Today there is a natural food renaissance bringing us back to nutritious and wholesome meals. Unprocessed, natural, organically grown, unaltered, pure and simple foods have become popular once again. Foods such as beans (legumes), greens, chicken, fish, cornmeal, pastas, brown rice, and whole-wheat breads to name a few, which were chosen by our ancestors for their nutritious, ethnic, and economic value, are back.

The resurgence of whole-food diets began when the medical community announced research findings that proved the positive effect of fiber on the digestive and intestinal tract. Other studies examined low-fat, high-fiber foods and their positive effects on the heart. Today the practice of using low-fat and high-fiber foods for the rehabilitation of diseases under the care of a physician or registered dietitian/nutritionist has found a place in mainstream society and has also become a popular option as a preventative health-care tool. As we live longer and the aging population steps into the twenty-first century, our quest to retain a youthful look and to feel good will strengthen our desire to examine our diet and continue the search for greater nutritional knowledge.

INTERNAL CLEANSING—THE BEAUTIFYING VALUE OF FIBER AND WATER

We are a society that likes to be clean. We take baths and showers; we wash our hands throughout the day; we cleanse our face every morning and night to remove makeup, dirt, and impurities. But when was the last time you thought about cleansing your intestines? Our digestive and intestinal tract has an extremely tough task from the moment food is placed in our mouth until our waste leaves our body. Ideally, the foods are metabolized as we eat them and are excreted on a day-to-day basis. Think of your intestinal tract like the plumbing system in your home. What happens to the pipes if you continually pour fat and debris down the drain? Eventually, the pipes become clogged and begin to back up. Well, the same thing happens to your intestines—not a pretty thought. A highly processed and low-fiber diet can cause the problem of irregularity. Please keep in mind that the speed at which food passes through our body has a direct relationship on how we feel and look. After the food has been metabolized and all the nutrients absorbed into our system, all that is left is toxic waste, and this waste should be eliminated daily. If this waste material hangs around too long in the lower intestine it becomes poisonous to our system. The American Cancer Society preaches the benefits of high-fiber and low-fat diets because it knows they have a direct influence on the prevention of colon cancer.

Where does fiber actually come from and how does it work? Every plant contains fiber because it is the component that helps to hold the plant together and hold water. This cellulose matter cannot be digested by humans because its composition cannot be broken down by the gastric juices in our stomach. This is the aspect of fiber that makes it so valuable and beneficial to our system. Its value is enhanced by drinking lots of water. Water and fiber mesh together causing an action that is similar to a large sponge or broom: They sweep away your body's waste and impurities. This action speeds up the excretion process, helping your intestines stay clean and in tiptop shape. When your digestive system works properly, nutrients are delivered quickly to your skin and free-radical toxins, which disrupt the healthy balance of your skin cells, are reduced. Naturally, a nutritious diet helps your complexion look healthier and it makes you feel better.

WATER—A PRECIOUS RENEWING FLUID FOR YOUR SKIN

Water is a precious fluid that is essential to good health. But most people don't take advantage of this natural, fat-free, and calorie-free therapeutic substance. Without an adequate water supply passing through our body each day we become "water deficient," causing a disorder called dehydration. When dehydration occurs there is not enough water to balance the fluids in our body. Basic bodily functions are affected and our purification system doesn't work efficiently, making it difficult to expel toxins. Water is also an essential nutrient for the skin; hydrated skin is soft and pliable; dehydrated skin looks parched and feels dry. But more important, your skin will reflect any of the internal inefficiencies that are caused by water deficiency.

How Much Water?

You may think you drink enough water each day, but you may be wrong if you're counting the wrong types of fluids. Coffee, tea, soda, beer, and pure fruit juice don't count. Coffee, tea, and beer act as diuretics so they are actually robbing your body of precious nutrients. All fluids on this list are loaded with negative nutrients such as caffeine, sugar, or artificial sweeteners that put stress on your system. It is vital to evaluate what you drink because water is more important than you could ever imagine.

The quantity of water you should consume each day is determined by how much you weigh. The recommended requirement for someone who is within 25 pounds of his or her ideal weight is eight, 8-ounce glasses of water a day. For every additional 25 pounds of excess weight, drink an extra 8-ounce glass of water.

What Happens If You Don't Drink Enough? When you don't drink enough water your body triggers a survival response that holds onto your water reserve, causing you to bloat and become swollen. The use of diuretics can give you temporary relief, but they can rob your skin of some valuable nutrients.

Ironically, the problem of retaining too much water can be resolved by drinking more water. When the body has a sufficient amount of water, it doesn't feel the need to conserve and releases the excess.

Water and Weight-loss Did you know that drinking plenty of water and weight loss go hand in hand? This is because of the way the kidney and the liver act as a purification system for your body. Without an adequate supply of water, your kidney has to work overtime. This in turn places undue stress on your liver because the liver now has to take care of the overflow of toxins from the kidneys. When the liver is overburdened like this, it can't function to its full capacity and therefore metabolizes less fat; this slows down the weight loss process. So not only does water consumption affect your complexion, it affects your entire appearance.

PROTECTING YOUR SKIN AGAINST FREE RADICALS

Free radicals and their effect on aging and the skin have had a great deal of publicity lately. The war against free radicals is a never-ending one because the catalysts for triggering the production of this hazard are all around us. But what exactly is this horror that is supposed to cause so much damage to our skin that it actually causes premature aging? These dangerous particles are actually microscopic molecules that have gone wild; you might say that the molecule is out of control. Each free radical is on a seek-and-destroy mission looking for healthy cells, and these "haywire" or "off balanced" molecules are usually found in groups of thousands. They do have the power to do extensive cell membrane damage as well as complete destruction to normal cells by robbing their oxygen.

What causes the development of free radicals? Smoking high-tar cigarettes, breathing in pollution, consuming fried foods and large quantities of alcohol can trigger the production of free radicals. Even the daily stress of life can lead to the production of free radicals. When your body is in a state of stress it produces extra adrenaline to help you through the crisis, but this increased metabolic state produces more free radicals. Ironically, individuals who are athletically inclined have been known to have higher levels of free radicals due to the higher oxygen consumption in the body.

Fortunately, our body has it own line of defense called "anti-oxidants" that protect us against this menace. But when the body is hit with the effects of repeated abuses (smoking cigarettes, alcohol consumption, daily stress, and eating plenty of fried foods) the natural reserve of anti-oxidants becomes depleted and the free radicals have a clear path to damage and destroy healthy cells.

The key to protecting your body and ultimately your skin against the damage that free radicals cause is to bump up your reserve of anti-oxidants. How can you fight back? Sports and spa nutritionist of the PGA National Resort & Spa, Cheryl Hartsough, R.D., L.D., recommends eating a diet that is full of anti-oxidants such as vitamins C and E, beta carotene, and selenium. These nutrients render the free radicals harmless before they damage the body's cells. These nutrients, combined with a high-complex carbo-

ANTI-OXIDANTS

Anti-oxidant: Beta Carotene

	Serving	*Amount*
Apricots	4 dried halves	2,500 IU
Asparagus	8 spears	1,500 IU
Cantaloupe	1/4 melon	3,400 IU
Carrot	1 raw	11,000 IU
Peach	1 med.	2,170 IU
Romaine lettuce	2 cups	1,100 IU
Spinach	1 cup, cooked	14,600 IU
Sweet Potato	1 small	8,100 IU

The USRDA (Recommended Daily Allowance) for vitamin A/beta carotene (beta carotene is the plant derivative) is 5,000 IU (International Units) per day for either a vitamin supplement and/or derived from a natural food source.

Anti-oxidant: Vitamin C

	Serving	*Amount*
Broccoli	1 cup	104 mg
Brussels Sprouts	1 cup	136 mg
Cabbage	1 cup	48 mg
Collard greens	1 cup	88 mg
Grapefruit	1 med.	76 mg
Orange Juice	6 oz.	90 mg
Strawberries	1 cup	132 mg

The USRDA for vitamin C is 60 milligrams, but the latest research shows that intake levels of 250–500 mg are quite safe and may be more effective in reducing your risk of disease.

Anti-oxidant: Vitamin E

	Serving	*Amount*
Almonds	1/4 cup	25 IU
100% whole-grain cereal	1 cup	.4 IU
100% whole-wheat bread	1 slice	.39 IU
Safflower oil	1 tbsp.	3.25 IU
Wheat Germ	1/4 cup	14 IU

The USRDA for vitamin E is 30 IU per day; however, research indicates that levels up to 200 IU may be more effective for the prevention of disease.

hydrate, low-fat (less than 20 percent), and high-fiber diet can counter these free radicals.

The preceding list of anti-oxidants will help you fight the war against free radicals and assist you in maintaining the integrity of cell structure, your health and ultimately the quality of your skin.

BALANCED EATING "EQUALS" A HEALTHY, MORE YOUTHFUL BODY AND SKIN

What is the magic formula for proper nutrition? The secret is not to get stuck on one food group because creating a balance (60 percent carbohydrates, 20 percent proteins, and no more than 20 percent fats) is obtained only when you consume a well-diversified collection of low-fat and high-fiber foods.

Moderation and variety are the key to balanced eating. Take it easy on the foods and seasonings that are on the "no-no" list such as ice cream, butter, margarine, red meats, alcoholic beverages, salt, and sugar to name just a few. Increase and vary foods known to offer nutritional components. Nutritional science is a young science and we are learning that there are a whole host of protective substances (phytochemicals) found in vegetables besides the well-recognized vitamins and minerals that we have known about.

Look at your diet. Are you eating the same thing day after day? Do you not vary your fruit, vegetable, and grain intake? Are you familiar with other grains besides rice and pasta? Just as you wouldn't even think of wearing the same clothes or outfit every day, you should not eat the same foods day in and day out.

Maximizing the effectiveness of your food intake may be easier than you think because there are plenty of foods that will help you maintain your energy level and the integrity of your body. Here are some of the many "power foods" that you could add to your menu repertoire. Kathie Swift, M.S., R.D., nutritionist at the Canyon Ranch Resort and Spa in Lenox, Massachusetts, recommends that you take a close look at the following list of power foods and nutrient-rich foods. These two tables will help guide you in your daily healthy food choices. Ms. Swift stresses the "variety element" is the key to healthy eating, and this philosophy is practiced every day at the Canyon Ranch.

WORDS YOU NEED TO KNOW

Anti-oxidant a compound that can help to neutralize or inactivate free radicals

Free radical a compound that can potentially damage human cells and start disease processes

Phytochemicals (phyto = plant; Greek) substances in plant foods in addition to vitamins and minerals, which exert protective effects

Carotenoids a yellow-orange pigment (phytochemical) in fruits and vegetables that may have protective properties against degenerative diseases; beta-carotene is just one of hundreds of carotenoids

TEN POWER FOOD CATEGORIES TO STREGTHEN YOUR SKIN

SOY

- Complete plant protein.
- Soy protein has two phytochemicals (Genistein and Isoflavones) that help with cancer and cardio protection.

tofu	tempeh	miso
soy milk	soy flour	soy nuts

CRUCIFEROUS VEGETABLES

- Excellent source of indoles, other phytochemicals that stimulate immune system's production of anti-cancer enzymes and anti-oxidants that help to neutralize free radicals.
- Cabbage, broccoli, brussels sprouts, cauliflower, kale, collards, mustard greens, rutabaga, turnip, arugala, watercress, radishes, horseradish.
- High in fiber, some very high in calcium.

ORANGE AND YELLOW FRUITS/VEGETABLES

- Excellent source of the pigment beta-carotene and other carotenoids, which act as antioxidants and can be very beneficial in the prevention of degenerative diseases (cataracts, heart disease, cancer, arthritis).
- Very easy to obtain protective levels through foods.

canteloupe	apricots	mangos	peaches
papayas	tangerines	nectarines	oranges
carrots	sweet potatoes	butternut squash	acorn squash

WHEAT BRAN/WHEAT GERM/WHOLE WHEAT

- Bran: high in insoluble fiber, extremely helpful for prevention of colon cancer, health of gastrointestinal tract; elimination.
- Wheat Germ: excellent source of vitamin E.
- Source of complex carbohydrates, low in fat, rich in both soluble and insoluble fiber, B-vitamins, and trace minerals.
- Refined grains lose approximately 80 percent of vitamins/minerals and retain only 25 percent of the fiber.

Amaranth	quinoa	millet	triticale	barley
buckwheat (kasha)	teff	bulgur	spelt	couscous

BEANS

- Good source of protein (incomplete, except soybean), low in fat, no cholesterol, good source of complex carbohydrates and B-vitamins.
- May help with blood-sugar control.
- High in fiber (soluble and insoluble), which can help alleviate gastrointestinal problems and lower LDL (bad) cholesterol.

split peas	kidney beans	pinto beans	black beans
chickpeas	white beans		

NUTS/SEEDS

- Excellent source of antioxidants, including vitamin E, selenium, and B-vitamins.

Nuts:	walnuts	chestnuts	peanuts	almonds	cashews
Seeds:	pumpkin	sunflower			

When you eat nuts and seeds think low quantity because they are high in quality. They are a rich source of essential fatty acids and an excellent source of the antioxidant vitamin E and mineral magnesium.

MUSHROOMS

- Good source of B-vitamins and copper.
- Shiitake, enoki, reishi, maltake show promise as immune-system boosters.
- Tea ear/wood ear act as anticoagulants to help keep the blood from clotting (helpful in heart disease).

GREENS/SEA VEGETABLES

- High in carotenoids and other phytochemicals, vitamins C and K, folic acid, iron, calcium, and fiber.
- Sea vegetables (wakame, nori, kombu, dulse) have a high mineral content including potassium, calcium, magnesium, iron, and iodine. Also high in fiber, vitamin C, and beta-carotene.

dandelion	mustard	beet greens	collard greens
kale	swiss chard	sorrel	broccoli rabe.

FISH

- Good source of protein, B-vitamins, and various minerals.
- Fattier fish (salmon, bass, carp, halibut, bluefish, herring, mackeral, rainbow trout, white fish) are excellent source of Omega-3 fatty acids (found in smaller amounts in shellfish and lean fish—flounder, sole, red snapper, haddock, cod, and canned tuna in water). Omega-3 fatty acids can help to increase HDL (good cholesterol) and may help to reduce inflammation in conditions such as arthritis, psoriasis, and inflammatory bowel disease.

NUTRIENT-RICH FOODS TO HELP YOUR SKIN LOOK HEALTHY

Beta Carotene

Apricots
Asparagus
Broccoli
Cantaloupe
Carrots
Endive
Greens
Mango
Papaya
Peach
Pumpkin
Red pepper
Spinach
Sweet potato
Tomato
Winter squash

B-1 Thiamine

Glucose is converted into energy via a compound known as pyruvic acid. Thiamin is responsible for ensuring that the pyruvic acid is fed into the energy cycle. If thiamine is absent the pyruvic acid builds up and causes an oxygen deficiency that results in loss of mental alertness, respiratory problems, and heart damage. B1 is also known as the growth vitamin and is usually part of natal multivitamins.

Baked potato with skin
Brewer's yeast
Oatmeal
Lentils
Pork loin
Rice Bran
Sunflower and sesame seeds
Wheat germ
Whole grains

B-2 Riboflavin

This vitamin is necessary for the production and repair of body tissue and appears to have a particular function in maintaining healthy mucous membrane. Riboflavin is also essential to efficient utilization of oxygen.

Almonds
Brewer's yeast
Broccoli
Chicken
Collard greens
Egg
Figs
Low-fat dairy products
Miso
Wheat germ
Whole grains

B-3 Niacin

Niacin improves blood circulation by dilating the blood vessels; it also reduces the cholesterol levels in the blood. Niacin is essential to the brain and nervous system and to maintaining a healthy skin, tongue, and digestive tract.

Avocado
Beef, lean
Bran
Brewer's yeast
Bulgur
Corn
Cream of Wheat
Mushrooms
Peanuts
Potato
Poultry
Salmon
Sunflower seeds
Tuna

B-6 Pyridoxine

Also known as an anti-depressant, B-6 is involved in more than 60 enzyme reactions in the body and is essential for sustaining life.

Banana
Carrots
Dark, leafy greens
Legumes
Mackerel
Potatoes
Poultry
Tuna
Wheat germ
Whole grains

B-12 Cobalamin

This vitamin does not occur in plants; it is found only in animal sources. Vitamin B-12 is essential to maintaining the myelin sheath, which is the coating that protects your nervous system.

Beef, lean
Chicken
Clams
Eggs
Fortified whole grains
Mackerel
Nonfat dairy
Salmon

Vitamin C

This water-soluble vitamin acts an antioxidant; by promoting absorption and the production of collagen (the connective tissue protein of the body), it helps the body resist bacterial and viral disease and produce anti-stress hormones.

Acerola cherries
Broccoli
Brussels sprouts
Cantaloupe
Citrus juice and fruit
Cranberry juice
Guava
Honeydew melon
Kiwi
Papaya
Peppers
Potato
Tomato

Vitamin E

This fat-soluble vitamin functions essentially as an antioxidant, helping to reduce the oxygen requirements of your body's organs and muscles and to regenerate your skin; acts as an anti-clotting agent, dissolves blood clots, and neutralizes the effect of harmful free radicals.

High fat	*Low fat*
Avocado	Fortified cereals
Corn oil	Greens
Margarine	Mango
Mayonnaise	Salmon
Nuts	Sweet potato
Sunflower seeds	Wheat germ
Wheat-germ oil	

Vitamin K

Vitamin K plays a role in blood coagulation or clotting.

Broccoli	Seaweed
Garbanzo beans	Spinach
Green tea	Turnip greens

Panthothenic acid

Pantothenic acid functions as a component of a co-enzyme, which is essential for energy production, for fat and cholesterol metabolism, for antibody formation and for a healthy nervous system.

Beef, lean	Mushrooms
Broccoli	Peanuts
Eggs	Rice bran
Haddock	Soybeans

Folacin

The vitamin folate (a form of a B vitamin) is required in the manufacturing process of new cells.

Asparagus	Oatmeal
Beets	Legumes
Broccoli	Orange juice
Brussels sprouts	Spinach
Corn	

Minerals

Boran

This trace mineral is active in the maintenance of human bone tissue and also may play a role in brain areas such as motor activity.

Apples
Broccoli
Carrots
Pears
Other fruits and vegetables
Soybean products

Calcium

The most abundant mineral in the body is calcium. Approximately 99 percent of it is found in our bones and teeth. The other 1 percent is found in our soft tissue. Calcium is essential to bone and tooth development, nerve action, heart and muscle action, and blood clotting. Calcium eases problems, menstrual cramps, and symptoms of menopause.

Corn tortillas
Figs, dried
Greens
Nonfat dairy
Orange juice, calcium fortified
Rhubarb
Salmon, with bones
Sardines, with bones
Sesame tahini
Skim-milk powder
Soy milk, calcium fortified
Tofu (amt. varies)

Chromium

This trace mineral works closely with hormone functions, insulin assisting in the glucose intake into the cells.

Apple with skin
Beef
Brewer's yeast
Broccoli
Corn
Fortified cereal
Peas
Sea scallops
Sole
Sweet potato
Wheat berries

Copper

This mineral activates an enzyme (cytochrome oxidase) that makes it possible for energy to be released to the cells.

Kidney beans
Lobster
Nuts
Oysters
Raisins
Sweet potato

Iron

This mineral is a component of hemoglobin; it helps carry oxygen through the blood stream and is very important for muscle tissue. At least 28 percent of the population is iron deficient.

- Bran cereals
- Cream of wheat
- Egg Yolk
- Legumes
- Meat
- Oatmeal
- Oysters
- Pumpkin seeds
- Spinach

Magnesium

This mineral is critical in the operation of enzymes in the body and directly affects the metabolism of potassium.

- Acorn squash
- Artichoke
- Broccoli
- Brown rice
- Figs
- Greens
- Miso
- Oatmeal
- Pumpkin seeds
- Quinoa
- Sunflower seeds
- Tofu

Manganese

This trace mineral is important to the digestive tract, the ligaments, and the development of bones and nerves. Manganese also serves to help your body better absorb vitamins B and C.

- Broccoli
- Carrots, boiled
- Green peas
- Peanuts
- Pineapple
- Rice bran
- Soybean products
- Spinach
- Walnuts
- Wheat bran
- Wheat germ
- Whole grains

Potassium

Potassium plays a major role in maintaining fluid electrolyte balance.

- Apricots, dried
- Baked potato
- Banana
- Blackstrap molasses
- Bran cereal
- Cantaloupe
- Figs
- Legumes
- Papaya
- Prunes
- Pumpkin
- Quinoa
- Skim milk
- Spinach
- Sweet potato
- Tomato sauce
- Winter squash

Selenium

Selenium used to be considered a poison, but recently it was found that the opposite was true. Recent studies have documented that selenium, along with vitamin E, acts as an antioxidant. The Food and Drug Administration (FDA) has recently acknowledged that selenium is essential and has indicated that up to 220 micrograms daily is safe.

Blackstrap molasses
Brazil nuts
Chicken
Kidney beans
Low-fat milk/yogurt
Mushrooms
Seafood
Sunflower seeds
Walnuts
Wheat germ
Whole grains

Zinc

This mineral is used to treat burns, alcoholism, sickle cell anemia, and acne. Zinc also aids in digestion and the healing process.

Beef
Bran
Fish
Legumes
Oysters
Poultry
Nuts and Seeds
Wheat bran/germ

Twenty Tips to Improve Your Skin Through Proper Nutrition

1. Drink water! At least 8 glasses a day.
2. Avoid fried foods. When using oils, try cold-pressed oils. Throw away any oil that has been in your cabinet for longer than six months. Oils should be refrigerated except for the small amount you may use in a week; keep in a small container.
3. Eat minimal sugar, chocolate, and potato chips, otherwise known as junk foods, which have little nutritional value.
4. Smoking increases wrinkles. If you can't kick the habit, consume extra amounts of vitamin C.
5. Watch your salt intake. Too much salt can lead to temporary swelling and puffiness.
6. Eat cooked egg whites . . . pure albumin protein.
7. The sulfur found in garlic, onions, and asparagus will aid in keeping the skin nice.

8. Vitamin E and aloe are very good to use topically on your skin.
9. Drink minimal amounts of alcohol.
10. Drink minimal amounts of soft drinks.
11. If you have a skin irritation and suspect a food allergy, eliminate suspected food and keep a food record to monitor your reaction.
12. Increase intake of raw vegetables. Not only high in fiber, but naturally higher in vitamins, phytochemicals, and enzymes than those that have been cooked, processed, or canned.
13. Thoroughly wash all food before it is eaten.
14. Eat all parts of fruits and vegetables. The white part inside the skin of citrus has vitamin C and bioflavinoids.
15. Have a cup of warm water with lemon juice in the morning.
16. When dining out eat broiled fishes, steamed or baked vegetables, and starches.
17. Eat little or no processed foods.
18. Eat food at a moderate pace. Food is energy, and if you eat food at a rapid pace you'll have more stress on your body, creating a stressful energy coming from your body. Stress creates stress. So pace yourself.
19. Get rid of your aluminum cooking utensils. Absolutely no benefit to the body.
20. Eat a high-fiber diet to cleanse the digestive track. Put a couple of tablespoons of wheat bran on your morning cereal; it has the bonus of extra B vitamins.

NUTRITIOUS EATING CAN BE FUN, BEAUTIFYING, AND SIMPLE

Do you ever feel as if you don't know what you want to eat? Have your meals become boring? Do you feel as if healthful eating deprives you of the foods you love? Eating properly for the health of your body and for your skin's health should not be a painful or mundane task. Use this section to help you turn your mealtime into an exciting adventure. Irresistible, yet simple and inexpensive recipes from the Canyon Ranch Resort and Spa in Lenox, Massachusetts, and Tucson, Arizona; PGA National Resort and Spa in Palm Beach

Gardens, Florida; and The Four Seasons Resort and Spa in Las Colinas, Texas can now grace your breakfast, lunch, and dinner table. Now you can learn how these famous spas serve sumptuous meals that are also healthful. Learn the tricks of creating delicious low-fat entrees in which fattening ingredients have been substituted with healthier options. Each of the following famous recipes has been presented in an easy step-by-step fashion with the nutritional facts listed so you can keep track of calories and your fat intake.

TEN SKIN-BEAUTIFYING RECIPES FROM THE CANYON RANCH SPA

As you can see from this sample menu, Canyon Ranch meals aren't what many think of as "spa food." This is real food, although you may find the serving sizes of protein and dessert items to be smaller than you usually eat. This supports the Canyon Ranch philosophy of "moderation, not deprivation." Keeping the portions of these higher calorie foods small (but large enough to be satisfying), allows you to spend more of your daily calorie allotment on complex carbohydrates such as whole-grain breads, pasta, potatoes, grains, and fruits and vegetables—the types of foods that have the fuel and fiber you need to run your body efficiently and keep you from feeling hungry between meals.

Canyon Ranch Weekend Menu

(This weekend menu can be used when you follow the plan in Chapter Five "Turn Your Home into a Spa for the Weekend.")

Friday

Dinner

	Calories	Fat Grams
*Broiled grouper with tarragon lime Sauce	225	1
Boiled red bliss potatoes (2 small)	80	Trace
with margarine (1 teaspoon)	35	4
Steamed broccoli (1/2 cup)	25	Trace
Nonfat frozen yogurt (1/3 cup)	80	Trace
Total	**445**	**5**

Saturday

Breakfast

	Calories	Fat Grams
*Hot oat cereal (1 cup)	155	3
with apricot sour cherry compote (2 teaspoon)	65	Trace
Total	**220**	**3**

Lunch

	Calories	Fat Grams
*Chicken fajita		
3 ounces marinated chicken	150	4
1 9-inch tortilla	120	4
*Canyon Ranch guacamole (2 T)	10	Trace
Light sour cream (2 T)	40	2
Bottled salsa (2 T)	10	Trace
Fresh Fruit (1/2 cup)	60	Trace
Total	**390**	**10**

Dinner

	Calories	Fat Grams
Mixed lettuce salad with nonfat bottled salad dressing	40	Trace
*Pasta alla Checca (2 cups pasta, 1/2 cup sauce)	495	6
Frozen fruit sorbet	100	Trace
Total	**635**	**6**
Total calories for the day	**1,245**	**24**

*Recipes: included for starred items
Trace = less than 1 gram

Sunday

Breakfast

	Calories	Fat Grams
*Sweet potato waffle (1/2 waffle)	180	5
Maple syrup (1 T)	50	1
1 cup cantaloupe, 1/4 cup blueberries, with 1/4 plain nonfat yogurt	100	Trace
Total	**330**	**6**

Lunch

	Calories	Fat Grams
Mixed green salad with nonfat bottled salad dressing	40	Trace
*Vegetarian pizza	255	7
Fresh sliced strawberries (1 cup)	60	Trace
Total	**355**	**7**

Dinner

	Calories	Fat Grams
Sliced cucumbers with nonfat bottled salad dressing	50	Trace
*Roulade of turkey with asparagus spears and crushed tomatoes	280	6
Brown rice (1/3 cup)	100	Trace
*Oatmeal crumb cake (1 slice)	135	5
Total	**565**	**11**
Total calories for the day	**1,250**	**24**

*Recipes: included for starred items
Trace = less than 1 gram

Recipes from the Canyon Ranch, Lenox, Massachusetts and Tucson, Arizona

Grouper with Tarragon Lime Sauce

1 pound grouper	1 tsp fructose
1 cup spinach	zest of one lime
1/2 cup parsley	1/4 tsp dried tarragon
2 tablespoons chopped shallots	1 tsp arrowroot powder
1/2 cup fish or chicken stock	1 tbsp evaporated skim milk

Cooking Directions

1. Divide grouper into 4 equal portions and set aside.
2. Blanch spinach and parsley by placing in a steamer basket over boiling water for 3 to 5 minutes. Transfer blanched spinach and parsley to a small piece of cheesecloth, gather up the ends and squeeze juice into a small bowl and discard spinach and parsley.
3. Prepare hot coals for grilling or preheat broiler.
4. Prepare lime zest by running zester over the peel, or grate colored portion of the rind. In a small saucepan, sauté shallots until translucent. Add stock, fructose, lime zest, and tarragon. Blend together arrowroot powder and evaporated skim milk and whisk into sauce. Simmer until desired thickness.
5. Grill or broil fish.
6. To serve, add reserved juice to sauce and ladle 2 tablespoons on each serving plate. Place fish in center of sauce.

Nutritional Facts

Makes 4 servings, each containing approximately:

225 calories	3 gm carbohydrates	1 gm fat
42 mg cholesterol	23 gm protein	69 mg sodium

Hot Cereal with Apricot and Sour Cherry Compote

8 pitted apricots, quartered, canned, or fresh (approx. 6 oz.)

1/4 teaspoon grated lemon zest

3/4 cup dried sour cherries 1 teaspoon honey

1 tablespoon lemon juice
1/4 cup water
2 cups uncooked quick oats
2 1/2 cups water

Cooking Directions

1. Combine apricots, cherries, lemon juice, 1/4 cup water, lemon zest, and honey in small sauté, pan and cook over medium heat for 2 minutes. Remove from heat and cool to room temperature.
2. Cook oats in remaining water according to directions on package. Divide oatmeal among 4 bowls and top with compote.

Nutritional Facts

Makes 4 servings, each containing approximately:

220 calories	45 gm carbohydrate	3 gm fat
0 mg cholesterol	7 gm protein	10 mg sodium

Chicken Fajita

4 skinned chicken breast halves, boned and defatted

Marinade:

2 tablespoons low-sodium soy sauce
4 whole-wheat tortillas
1/4 teaspoon minced ginger root
1 1/3 cups Canyon Ranch guacamole (see recipe)
1/4 teaspoon minced garlic
1 cup bottled salsa
2 tablespoons olive oil
1/2 cup commercial light sour cream
1/3 cup finely chopped cilantro
pinch chili powder
3 tablespoons beer
1/2 teaspoon Tabasco sauce
1/2 orange, thinly sliced
1/2 lemon, thinly sliced
1/2 lime, thinly sliced
1 tablespoon chopped parsley

Cooking Directions

1. Combine marinade ingredients in a shallow baking dish and mix well.
2. Cover chicken breasts with marinade, turning to coat evenly. Cover and refrigerate for at least 2 hours or as long as overnight.
3. Prepare hot coals for grilling or preheat broiler.
4. Lift chicken breasts from marinade and grill or broil 3 to 4 minutes per side. Cut chicken into strips and serve with whole-wheat tortilla, salsa, guacamole, and light sour cream.

Nutritional Facts

Makes 4 servings, each containing approximately:

340 calories*	27 gm carbohydrate	11 gm fat
86 mg cholesterol	34 gm protein	508 mg sodium

*Calories will vary somewhat depending on the brand of bottled salsa you use.

Canyon Ranch Guacamole

1/2 pound frozen asparagus spears, approx. one small package

1/8 teaspoon chili powder

1 1/2 teaspoons lemon juice

pinch cumin

2 tablespoons chopped onion

pinch black pepper

1/2 cup finely diced tomato

1/3 teaspoon minced garlic

1/3 teaspoon salt (optional)

dash Tabasco sauce

2 tablespoons commercial light sour cream

Cooking Directions

1. Defrost and lightly steam asparagus spears.
2. Combine all ingredients in a blender and whirl until smooth.
3. Refrigerate several hours or overnight before serving.

Nutritional Facts

Makes 6 servings, each containing approximately:

25 calories	4 gm carbohydrate	Trace fat
4 gm cholesterol	2 gm protein	220 mg sodium

Alla Checca Sauce for Pasta

4 cups diced ripe plum tomatoes, about 4 medium

1/2 cup chopped fresh parsley

1/2 teaspoon salt

2 teaspoons extra virgin olive oil

2 teaspoons minced garlic

1/4 teaspoon freshly ground black pepper

1/2 cup chopped fresh basil leaves

1/4 teaspoon crushed red pepper

Cooking Directions

1. Bring large pot of water to a boil. Cut a shallow *X* in the blossom end of the tomatoes with a sharp knife. Drop the tomatoes into the boiling water for 2 minutes, then transfer to a bowl of cold water. The skins should peel off easily.
2. Chop peeled tomatoes. You should have about 4 cups.
3. Sprinkle diced tomatoes with the salt and mix well. Place tomatoes in a colander and allow to drain.
4. Combine the minced garlic, chopped basil, parsley, olive oil, black pepper, and red pepper in a medium sauce pan. Add the drained tomatoes and heat until warm. Serve over pasta.

Nutritional Facts

Makes 6 (1/2 cup) servings, each containing approximately:

75 calories	7 gm carbohydrates	5 gm fat
0 mg cholesterol	2 gm protein	212 mg sodium

Sweet Potato Waffle

3/4 cup peeled, cooked, and mashed sweet potatoes (about 1/2 pound raw)

3/4 cup 2% milk

1 1/2 teaspoons melted margarine

1/2 cup whole-wheat flour

1 medium egg white, slightly beaten

1 teaspoon baking powder

1/4 teaspoon salt

Cooking Directions

1. Preheat waffle iron
2. In a large bowl, combine cooked sweet potatoes, margarine, egg white, and milk. Beat until blended. Add flour, baking powder, and salt. Stir until smooth.
3. Spray waffle iron with nonstick vegetable coating.
4. Pour 3/4 cup of batter onto center of waffle iron and bake.

Nutritional Facts

Makes 4 (1/2-waffle) servings, each containing approximately:

180 calories	33 gm carbohydrates	3 gm fat
4 mg cholesterol	6 gm protein	255 mg sodium

Pizza Crust

(Don't try to eliminate the salt in this recipe—it's necessary for the dough to rise properly.)

1/2 ounce yeast

1 cup warm water

3/4 cup white flour

1 1/2 cups whole-wheat flour

2 teaspoons olive oil

1/4 teaspoon salt

2 teaspoons cornmeal

Cooking Directions

1. Soften yeast in the warm water in a medium bowl. Add white flour and mix well. Add olive oil and salt. Stir until well mixed.
2. Add whole-wheat flour. Turn out on a floured board and knead, about 10 to 15 minutes, until smooth and elastic.
3. Rub the inside of a large bowl lightly with vegetable oil. Put dough in bowl and turn so the oiled side is up. Cover dough with waxed paper or plastic wrap and place in a warm spot for 1 1/2 to 2 hours until the dough is doubled

in bulk. Punch down and knead a few times. Re-form into a ball and refrigerate until cold, 20 to 30 minutes.

4. Divide the dough in half and roll out on a lightly floured board. Sprinkle 2 12-inch pizza pans with teaspoon cornmeal each, and transfer crusts to pans. If you are not going to make the pizzas immediately, wrap and freeze. Thaw out completely before placing the sauce and toppings and cheese over the top. (See the recipe for Pizza.)

Nutritional Facts

Makes 12 servings, each containing approximately:

130 calories	24 gm carbohydrates	1 gm fat
0 mg cholesterol	5 gm protein	77 mg sodium

Pizza

Before you begin this recipe, make the pizza crust (see previous recipe). Crush the dried basil and oregano with a mortar and pestle for optimum flavor.

Sauce:

1/2 chopped onion
1 garlic clove, crushed
1/4 cup finely chopped parsley
2 tablespoons vegetable stock or water
1 (8 oz) can tomato paste
1 teaspoon crushed oregano
1/2 teaspoon crushed basil
1/2 teaspoon salt (optional)
1/4 teaspoon freshly ground black pepper

Topping:

1 large, thinly sliced onion
1 cup thinly sliced mushrooms
1/2 small green pepper, sliced
1/2 small red pepper, sliced
1 1/4 cups thinly sliced zucchini
6 ounces shredded part-skim mozzarella cheese
1 pizza crust (see recipe)

Cooking Directions

1. Make pizza crust.
2. Preheat oven to 425 degrees
3. Sauté the onion, garlic, and parsley in the vegetable stock in a small saucepan until soft. Remove from heat and add

tomato paste, oregano, basil, salt, and black pepper and mix thoroughly.

4. Spread the sauce over pizza crust. Arrange the onions, mushrooms, pepper slices and zucchini decoratively on top of the sauce. Bake in the preheated oven on the lowest shelf for 10 minutes. Remove from oven.
5. Place the shredded cheese on the pizza and bake for an additional 5 minutes or until bottom is lightly browned. If the pizza begins to brown too much before the crust is done place a square of aluminum foil over the top and continue to bake until the bottom crust is lightly browned. Remove from oven. Allow to stand for 3 to 5 minutes before slicing. Cut pizza into 6 slices.

Nutritional Facts

Makes 6 servings, each containing (including crust) approximately:

225 calories	38 gm carbohydrates	7 gm fat
16 mg cholesterol	14 gm protein	573 mg sodium

Roulade of Turkey with Asparagus and Crushed Tomatoes

1 pound skinned turkey breast, boned and defatted

2 tablespoons chicken stock	1/4 teaspoon basil
12 small asparagus spears	1/4 teaspoon oregano
2 tablespoons diced chives	1/4 teaspoon minced garlic
1 tablespoons olive oil	pinch pepper
1 tablespoon shallots	pinch cayenne

4 medium tomatoes, peeled and diced (approx. 5 cups)

Cooking Directions

1. Cut turkey breast diagonally on the bias into 4 equal portions
2. Place turkey breast slices between two sheets of clear wrap and flatten with meat mallet to about 1/4-inch thick. Cut 4 pieces of clear wrap double the size of the flattened breast, lay each breast on a piece, and set aside.
3. Place asparagus spears in a collapsible steamer basket over boiling water and steam for 3 minutes. Transfer into bowl and toss with chives.

4. Lay 3 asparagus spears parallel in center of each flattened breast. Roll breast around each asparagus to form roulade. Wrap breasts individually in plastic wrap and close tightly. Poke small hole in wrap for venting. Set aside.
5. In heavy saucepan, sauté shallots in olive oil. Add tomatoes, chicken stock, and seasoning. Cook for 5 minutes.
6. In medium saucepan, heat 2 cups water just to the point of boiling. Turn down heat and drop roulades into water and cook 6 to 8 minutes. Lift roulades out of the water and unwrap. Cut into 3 pieces and fan out over 1/4 cup crushed tomatoes.

Nutritional Facts

Makes 4 servings, each containing approximately:

200 calories	8 gm carbohydrates	6 gm fat
8 mg cholesterol	29 gm protein	85 mg sodium

Oatmeal Crumb Cake

2/3 cup all-purpose flour
2/3 cup whole-wheat pastry flour
1/4 cup oat bran
1/2 cup fructose
1/4 cup canola oil
1/4 cup rolled oats
1/2 teaspoon cinnamon
2 1/4 teaspoons baking powder
2/3 cup evaporated skim milk
2 egg whites, slightly beaten
1/2 teaspoon nutmeg
2 tablespoons finely chopped hazelnuts

Cooking Directions

1. Preheat oven to 350° F. Spray bread pan with nonstick vegetable coating.
2. In small mixing bowl, combine flours, oat bran, fructose, and oil. Mix well.
3. Prepare crumb topping by removing 1/4 cup flour mixture and combine with rolled oats, nuts, nutmeg, and cinnamon in a small bowl and set aside.
4. Add baking powder, milk, and egg to remaining flour mixture and mix well.

5. Pour 1/2 of the batter into prepared bread pan. Sprinkle 1/2 of the topping mixture over, then repeat step with remaining batter and topping.
6. Bake in preheated oven for 25 minutes or until cake is lightly browned.

Nutritional Facts

Makes 16 servings, each containing approximately:

130 calories	18 gm carbohydrates	5 gm fat
Trace cholesterol	3 gm protein	85 mg sodium

Twenty-Seven Recipes fom the PGA National Resort and Spa

PGA Nutrition Philosophy The goal of the PGA National Resort and Spa, Palm Beach Gardens, Florida, is to teach individuals how to make healthy food choices and to achieve optimal health and well-being through responsible weight management. The philosophy of the PGA "Spa Cuisine Program" is based on sound nutritional principles from the latest scientific research that *total* calories are not the most important issue. In other words, all calories are not equal—fat calories count more. Any cuisine from around the world can be made healthier by substituting low-fat products for their higher-fat counterparts. Nutritionist Cheryl Hartsough, R.D., L.D., has created each of the following recipes to meet specific nutritional goals exclusively for the PGA National Resort and Spa in Palm Beach Gardens, Florida.

SOUPS

Longhorn Gazpacho

Ingredients

3 cups low-sodium vegetable-juice cocktail

1/4 cup diced green bell pepper

1/4 diced cucumber

4 tomatillas, diced

2 red tomatoes, diced

2 tablespoons lime juice

2 yellow tomatoes, diced

1 tablespoon minced garlic

1/2 cup cooked or canned black beans, rinsed

1 tablespoon cilantro, chopped

1/2 cup diced red onion

hot pepper sauce to taste

Cooking Directions

In large bowl stir all ingredients; cover and refrigerate at least 2 hours.

Nutritional Facts

Makes 8 (1 cup) servings, each containing:

calories: 65	protein: 3 g
fat: 0 g	sodium: 38 mg
cholesterol: 0 mg	fiber: 2 g
carbohydrate: 14 g	calcium: 30 mg

0% fat 86% carbohydrate 14% protein

Butternut Squash Soup

Ingredients

4 cups low-sodium chicken stock, skimmed

2 sprigs fresh or 1 tbsp dried rosemary

1 1/2 pound fresh butternut squash, peeled, seeded, and cut into chunks

2 sprigs fresh or 1 tbsp dried marjoram

1 pound green apples, cored and chopped

1/4 teaspoon salt

1/2 pound yellow onion (about 2 medium), peeled and chopped

1/4 teaspoon black pepper

1 teaspoon lemon juice

Cooking Directions

1. In large saucepot or Dutch oven over medium heat bring all ingredients to a boil.

2. Reduce heat; cover and simmer 30 minutes until squash is tender.
3. In blender at high speed puree mixture in several batches until smooth. (Care should be taken to follow manufacturer's directions for processing hot liquids.)

Nutritional Facts

Makes 12 (3/4 cup) servings, each containing:

calories: 68	protein: 1 g
fat: 0.6 g	sodium: 52 mg
cholesterol: 0 mg	fiber: 2 g
carbohydrate: 15 g	calcium: 28 mg

7% fat 88% carbohydrate 5% protein

Chilled Tropical Fruit Soup

Ingredients

30 strawberries, divided

1 tablespoon honey

1/2 medium cantaloupe, peeled and cut into pieces

1/2 cup ginger ale

1/2 pineapple, peeled and cut into pieces

alfalfa sprouts for garnish

1 banana, peeled and sliced

3 coconuts, cut in half, optional*

1/2 cup orange juice

6 mint sprigs for garnish

Cooking Directions

1. Cut 6 strawberries into quarters and 18 strawberries into fans; set aside.
2. In blender combine remaining 6 strawberries, cantaloupe, pineapple, banana, orange juice, and honey; blend until smooth.
3. Add ginger ale.

To serve: On each of 6 plates place bed of alfalfa sprout, top with coconut half or soup bowl; fill with 1/6 fruit soup. Float 4 strawberry quarters in each bowl.

Garnish plate with strawberry fans and mint.

*Ask butcher to saw coconuts in half; reserve coconut milk for another use.

Nutritional Facts

Makes 6 servings, each containing:

calories: 113	protein: 2 g
fat: 0 g	sodium: 8 mg
cholesterol: 0 mg	fiber: 4 g
carbohydrate: 27 g	calcium: 29 mg

0% fat 95% carbohydrate 5% protein

Vegetable Harvest Soup

Ingredients

- 1 carrot, peeled and diced
- 1 rib celery, diced
- 1/2 medium onion, peeled and diced
- 1/2 zucchini, diced
- 1 tablespoon minced garlic
- 1 teaspoon olive oil
- 1 cup diced fresh pumpkin
- 1/2 yellow squash, diced
- 1 tablespoon chopped cilantro or parsley
- 1/2 cup whole-kernel corn
- 1/2 cup wild rice, cooked
- 3 plum tomatoes, diced
- 5 cups low-sodium vegetable broth, skimmed

Cooking Directions

1. In large saucepan or Dutch oven over medium heat sauté carrot, celery, onion, garlic, and cilantro in oil and 2 tbsp. vegetable stock until onion is translucent.
2. Add remaining vegetables; sauté 3 minutes more, stirring occasionally.
3. Add remaining vegetable broth; bring to a boil.
4. Reduce heat to low; simmer 30 minutes.
5. Stir in wild rice.

Nutritional Facts

Makes 6 (1 1/2) servings, each containing:

calories: 85	protein: 2.5 g
fat: 2 g	sodium: 23 mg
cholesterol: 0 mg	fiber: 2 g
carbohydrate: 15 g	calcium: 27 mg

20% fat 70% carbohydrate 10% protein

SALADS

Hot Spinach Salad

Ingredients

1/4 cup thinly sliced red onion

1/3 cup balsamic vinegar

1 tablespoon chopped garlic

1 roasted red pepper, cut into strips

1 tablespoon olive oil

1/2 cup snow peas, sliced crosswise in thirds

3/4 cup sliced mushrooms

1 pound fresh spinach, trimmed and washed

Cooking Directions

1. In medium skillet over high heat sauté onion and garlic in oil 2 minutes.
2. Add mushrooms and vinegar.
3. Reduce heat to low; simmer until mushrooms and onions are tender.
4. Add roasted pepper and snow peas.
5. Cook over high heat 1 minute.
6. Remove from heat and toss with spinach in large bowl until well coated.

Serve immediately on warm plates.

Nutritional Facts

Makes 2 servings, each containing:

calories: 160	protein: 7 g
fat: 7 g	sodium: 184 mg
cholesterol: 0 mg	fiber: 11 g
carbohydrate: 18 g	calcium: 257 mg

38% fat 45% carbohydrate 17% protein

Carrot Raisin Salad

This vitamin-A rich salad is great for a picnic.

Ingredients

1/2 cup plain nonfat yogurt

1/2 cup canned crushed pineapple in pineapple juice

2 tablespoons reduced-calorie mayonnaise

2 tbsp. raisins

1 teaspoon sugar (optional)

2 tsp. shredded coconut

1 pound carrots, peeled and grated (2 1/2 cups)

Cooking Directions

1. In large bowl beat yogurt, mayonnaise, and sugar until blended.
2. Add carrots, pineapple, and raisins.
3. Toss to coat well.
4. Refrigerate.
5. Just before serving toss again; sprinkle with coconut.

Nutritional Facts

Makes 6 (1/2 cup) servings, each containing:

calories: 78	protein: 2 g
fat: 1.8 g	sodium: 71 mg
cholesterol: 2 g	fiber: 2.5 g
carbohydrate: 14 g	calcium: 63 mg

20% fat 71% carbohydrate 9% protein

VEGETABLES

Sautéed Cabbage

Ingredients

2 tablespoons rice wine vinegar

2 tablespoons low-sodium soy sauce

3 cups shredded Chinese cabbage

2 teaspoons cornstarch

1 teaspoon sugar

2 drops hot chili oil, optional

2 teaspoons sesame oil

2 cups shredded green cabbage

2 cups shredded red cabbage

1/4 cup chicken stock

3 cloves garlic, minced

2 tablespoons sesame seeds

Cooking Directions

1. In small bowl stir vinegar, soy sauce, sesame oil, cornstarch, sugar, and chili oil; set aside.
2. In large nonstick skillet or Dutch oven over medium heat sauté cabbages in chicken stock 5 minutes until tender, stirring occasionally.
3. Add soy sauce mixture; cook 1 minute more, tossing to coat evenly.
4. Sprinkle with sesame seeds.

Nutritional Facts

Makes 6 servings, each containing:
calories: 57
fat: 3 g
cholesterol: 0 mg
carbohydrate: 6 g
protein: 2 g
sodium: 192 mg
fiber: 0.8 g
calcium: 67 mg
44% fat 42% carbohydrate 14% protein

Twice Baked Potatoes

Ingredients

2 large Idaho potatoes (8 oz. each), washed

2 green onions, chopped

1/2 cup 1% fat cottage cheese
1 tablespoon chopped fresh or 1 tsp. dried parsley
3 tablespoons grated Parmesan cheese
1 tablespoon chopped fresh or 1 tsp. dried basil
1 small onion, diced
1/2 teaspoon ground white pepper
1 clove garlic, minced
1/4 teaspoon ground red pepper (cayenne)
2 teaspoons olive oil
1 teaspoon paprika
3/4 package (10 oz.) frozen chopped spinach, thawed and drained

Cooking Directions

1. In a 400° F. oven bake pierced potatoes 1 hour until fork-tender. Cool.
2. Cut in half lengthwise; scoop out flesh leaving 1/2″ shell. Set shell aside.
3. Preheat oven to 350° F.
4. In medium bowl mash scooped potato with cheeses.
5. In large skillet over medium heat sauté onion and garlic in oil until onion is translucent.
6. Add spinach; cook 2 minutes.
7. Add spinach-onion mixture, green onions, parsley, basil, and peppers to mashed potato mixture. Beat until well combined.
8. Spoon or pipe potato mixture into reserved potato shells.
9. Bake 15 minutes until top is lightly brown and crispy.

Nutritional Facts

Makes 4 servings, each containing:
calories: 193
fat: 4 g
cholesterol: 3 mg
carbohydrate: 31 g
protein: 9 g
sodium: 117 mg
fiber: 4 g
calcium: 162 mg
18% fat 64% carbohydrate 18% protein

ENTRÉES

Grilled Honey Basil Chicken

Ingredients

6 boneless, skinless chicken breast halves (4 oz. each)

Marinade:

2 cups raspberry vinegar

6 tablespoons fresh chopped or 6 tsp. dried basil

6 tablespoons Dijon mustard

1 teaspoon ground black pepper

1/4 cup low-sodium soy sauce

1 teaspoon dried thyme

1/4 cup honey

Cooking Directions

1. In large saucepan stir all marinade ingredients until well combined.
2. Add chicken.
3. Refrigerate 1 hour to blend flavors.
4. Spray grill rack or broiler pan with cooking spray; set aside.
5. Preheat grill or broiler.
6. Remove chicken, reserving remaining marinade.
7. Grill or broil chicken about 15–20 minutes until cooked through.
8. Heat reserved marinade to boiling. Cook until reduced by half; serve over chicken.

Nutritional Facts

Makes 6 servings, each containing:

calories: 202
fat: 2 g
cholesterol: 68 mg
carbohydrate: 18 g
9% fat 35% carbohydrate 56% protein

protein: 28 g
sodium: 597 mg
fiber: 0 g
calcium: 44 mg

Smoked Turkey Quesadilla

Ingredients

4 whole-wheat flour tortillas (8″ each)

1 cup Black Bean Relish (see recipe)

1/2 cup shredded part-skim mozzarella cheese

1/2 cup Spa Avocado Salsa (see recipe)

8 ounces skinless, boneless smoked turkey, diced

1/2 cup nonfat sour cream

2 cups shredded greens

Cooking Directions

For each quesadilla:

1. In 9″ skillet over high heat place a tortilla.
2. Sprinkle with 2 tablespoons cheese and 1/4 portion of diced turkey.
3. Cook until cheese melts.
4. Fold in half and remove from pan.

To serve: Cut each quesadilla in thirds. On each of 4 plates place 1/2 cup greens, top with cut quesadilla, 1/4 cup relish, 2 tablespoons salsa and 2 tablespoons sour cream.

Nutritional Facts

Makes 4 servings, each containing:

calories: 345	protein: 31 g
fat: 9 g	sodium: 206 mg
cholesterol: 66 mg	fiber: 4 g
carbohydrate: 34 g	calcium: 256 mg

23.5% fat 40% carbohydrate 36% protein

Spa Avocado Salsa

Ingredients

4 medium tomatoes, diced

2 tablespoons lemon juice

1 large avocado, seeded, peeled, and diced

2 tablespoons chopped fresh cilantro

1/4 cup diced red onion

1 tablespoons minced garlic

Cooking Directions

In medium bowl gently stir all ingredients until combined. Refrigerate at least 1 hour to blend flavors.

Nutritional Facts

Makes 24 (2-T) servings, each containing:

calories: 20	protein: 0.5 g
fat: 1.1 g	sodium: 3 mg
cholesterol: 0 mg	fiber: 0.5 g
carbohydrate: 2 g	calcium: 4 mg

50% fat 40% carbohydrate 10% protein

Black Bean Relish

Ingredients

1 cup cooked or canned black beans, rinsed and drained

2 tablespoons low-sodium chicken stock or broth, skimmed

1/4 cup thawed frozen or vacuum-packed canned whole-kernel corn

1 tablespoon chopped cilantro

1/4 cup diced seeded tomato

1 tablespoon minced garlic

2 tablespoons lime juice

Cooking Directions

1. In small bowl stir all ingredients until well blended.
2. Cover and refrigerate at least 1 hour to blend flavors.

Nutritional Facts

Makes 8 (1/4 cup) servings, each containing:

calories: 44	protein: 2 g
fat: 0.5 g	sodium: 3 mg
cholesterol: 0 mg	fiber: 1 g
carbohydrate: 8 g	calcium: 16 mg

10% fat 72% carbohydrate 18% protein

Guava BBQ Shrimp

Ingredients

1 pound large shrimp (16–20), peeled and deveined
1/2 cup Pineapple Teriyaki Sauce (see recipe)
1/2 cup Guava BBQ Sauce (see recipe)
4 cups torn salad greens
2 cups cooked cellophane noodles
1 cup Banana Salsa (see recipe)
1/2 cup julienne red bell pepper

Cooking Directions

1. In medium saucepan stir shrimp and Guava BBQ Sauce; let stand 30 minutes.
2. Preheat grill or broiler.
3. Lightly drain shrimp, reserving extra BBQ sauce.
4. Grill or broil shrimp until done, turning constantly.
5. Meanwhile, in large skillet over medium-high heat stir-fry cellophane noodles, pepper, and Pineapple Teriyaki Sauce until pepper is tender-crisp.
6. Heat reserved BBQ sauce to boiling.

To serve: On each of 4 plates place 1 cup salad greens topped with 1/4 noodle mixture alongside 1/4 Banana Salsa topped with 1/4 serving shrimp. Just before serving brush shrimp with heated BBQ sauce.

Nutritional Facts

Makes 4 servings, each containing:
calories: 308
fat: 2 g
cholesterol: 135 mg
carbohydrate: 51 g
protein: 19 g
sodium: 682 mg
fiber: 1 g
calcium: 75 mg
8% fat 67% carbohydrate 25% protein

Guava B-B-Q Sauce

Ingredients

1/4 cup ketchup
1 tablespoon guava puree
1 tablespoon cider vinegar
1/2 tablespoon honey
1 teaspoon brown sugar
1/2 teaspoon jerk seasoning*
1/2 teaspoon vegetable oil

Cooking Directions

1. In small bowl whisk all ingredients until well blended.
2. Store covered in refrigerator up to 4 weeks.

*Jerk seasoning is available in the spice section of your supermarket or specialty food store. If not available, substitute mixture of teaspoon each of Worcestershire sauce, allspice, cinnamon, sugar, garlic powder, scallion, ground pepper, and Tabasco sauce to taste.

Nutritional Facts

Makes 4 (2-T) servings, each containing:
calories: 38
fat: 0.4 g
cholesterol: 0 mg
carbohydrate: 8.5 g
protein: 0.2 g
sodium: 179 mg
fiber: 0 g
calcium: 7 mg
9% fat 89% carbohydrate 2% protein

Banana Salsa

Ingredients

1/3 cup diced banana
1/3 cup diced seeded tomato
1/4 cup diced red onion
2 tablespoons cider vinegar
1 tablespoon brown sugar
1 teaspoon chopped cilantro

Cooking Directions

1. In small bowl gently stir all ingredients until well combined.
2. Cover and refrigerate at least 1 hour to blend flavors.

Nutritional Facts

Makes 4 (2-T) servings, each containing:

calories: 35	protein: 0 g
fat: 0 g	sodium: 2 mg
cholesterol: 0 mg	fiber: 0.8 g
carbohydrate: 9 g	calcium: 6 mg

0% fat 100% carbohydrate 0% protein

Pineapple Teriyaki Sauce

Ingredients

vegetable cooking spray

1/4 cup lite soy sauce

1 clove garlic, minced

2 tablespoons chopped fresh or 2 teaspoons dried basil

1/2 cup unsweetened pineapple juice

1/2 tablespoon cornstarch

1/2 cup chopped fresh or canned crushed pineapple

Cooking Directions

1. Spray medium saucepan with cooking spray.
2. Add garlic.
3. Cook over medium-high heat 1 minute.
4. Add remaining ingredients; bring to a boil, stirring.
5. Reduce heat to low; simmer 5 minutes, stirring occasionally.

Nutritional Facts

Makes 5 (1/4-cup) servings, each containing:

calories: 41	protein: 1.5 g
fat: 0 g	sodium: 744 mg
cholesterol: 0 mg	fiber: 0 g
carbohydrate: 9 g	calcium: 16 mg

0% fat 88% carbohydrate 12% protein

Basil & Tomato Quiche

Ingredients

vegetable cooking spray
3/4 cup shredded mozzarella cheese
24 egg whites (1 cup of egg substitute)
2 tablespoons grated Parmesan cheese
2 whole eggs
2 tablespoons chopped green onion
1/4 cup canned evaporated skim milk
1/2 clove garlic, minced
2 large tomatoes, peeled, seeded, and diced
pinch ground white pepper
8 fresh basil leaves, chopped
pinch ground nutmeg

Cooking Directions

1. Preheat oven to 350° F.
2. Spray 8″ by 8″ glass baking dish with cooking spray, set aside.
3. In large bowl beat eggs with milk; stir in remaining ingredients until well combined.
4. Pour into prepared pan.
5. Bake 30 minutes until knife inserted into center comes out clean.

Nutritional Facts

Makes 8 servings, each containing:
calories: 140
fat: 5 g
cholesterol: 73 mg
carbohydrate: 6 g
protein: 18 g
sodium: 296 mg
fiber: 0.5 g
calcium: 201 mg
32% fat 16% carbohydrate 52% protein

Crab Papaya Avocado Salad over Greens

Ingredients

3 papayas

2 cups lump crab meat, rinsed and drained

Juice of 1 lime

1 shallot, finely chopped

3 tablespoons golden raisins

1 cup Spa Avocado Salsa (see recipe)

6 cups torn salad greens

Cooking Directions

1. Cut papayas in half; remove seeds and scoop out flesh; set shells aside.
2. Dice flesh.
3. In large bowl gently mix diced papayas, crab meat, lime juice, shallot, and raisins.
4. Add Spa Avocado Salsa.
5. Toss until well combined.

To serve: On each of 6 plates place 1 cup salad greens topped with a papaya half filled with 1/6 crab salad.

Nutritional Facts

Makes 6 servings, each containing:
calories: 170
fat: 2.5 g
cholesterol: 40 mg
carbohydrate: 20 g
protein: 17 g
sodium: 493 mg
fiber: 2.5 g
calcium: 85 mg
13% fat 47% carbohydrate 40% protein

Tacckino Primavera

Ingredients

Pasta:

8 ounces white turkey or chicken meat, roasted without skin

1 red pepper, chopped

6 cups cooked small pasta shells (sea shells or bow ties)

1/2 cup celery, chopped

2 cups chopped tomato

1/4 cup red onion, diced

1 zucchini, chopped

4 ounces sliced mushrooms

2 ounces sliced black olives

1/2 cup leeks, chopped

1/4 cup sundried tomatoes, soaked in coffee and water, then boiled and drained

Dressing:

1 tablespoon olive oil

4 tablespoons chopped parsley

1 teaspoon mustard powder

2 tablespoon grated Parmesan cheese

1/2 cup chicken broth, nonfat

1/2 teaspoon white pepper

1/4 cup chopped basil

4 garlic cloves, chopped

pinch red pepper flakes

1 teaspoon Worcestershire sauce

2 ounces balsamic vinegar

Cooking Directions:

1. Place all the pasta ingredients in a large bowl.
2. Toss together the dressing ingredients and add to pasta mixture.
3. Chill 1 hour before serving.

Serve over leafy greens.

Nutritional Facts

Makes six, 2-cup servings, each containing:

Calories: 270 Fat grams: 4

LOW CALORIE DESSERT AND SNACKS

Energy Bar

Ingredients

vegetable cooking spray
4 ounces dried apricots, finely chopped
3 cups puffed rice cereal
1/2 cup honey
1 cup puffed wheat cereal
1/2 cup unprocessed bran
1 1/2 cups regular or quick rolled oats (not instant)
1/2 cup thawed frozen unsweetened apple juice concentrate
1/2 cup raisins
3 tablespoons light corn syrup
2 tablespoons molasses
1 teaspoon ground cinnamon
2 tablespoons dry sesame seeds

Cooking Directions

1. Preheat oven to 275° F.
2. Spray 11″ x 17″ baking pan with cooking spray; set aside.
3. In large bowl with wooden spoon mix apricots and next 10 ingredients for 5 minutes until well combined.
4. Turn into prepared pan; flatten with spatula, pushing down hard.
5. Sprinkle with sesame seeds; flatten again.
6. Bake 50 minutes (for chewy texture) to 1 hour.
7. Cool on wire rack 10 minutes. With very sharp knife cut into 15 bars (5 columns by 3 rows).

To store: Tightly wrap individually in foil. Store up to 1 week. Freeze for longer storage.

Nutritional Facts

Makes 15 bars, each containing:
calories: 157
fat: 1 g
cholesterol: 0 mg
carbohydrate: 35 g
5% fat 89% carbohydrate 6% protein
protein: 2.5 g
sodium: 10 mg
fiber: 3 g
calcium: 38 mg

Strawberry Smoothie

Ingredients

1 1/2 cups strawberries, hulled and cut in half

1/2 cup vanilla nonfat yogurt

2 ripe medium bananas, frozen and cut into pieces

1 tablespoon honey

8 ice cubes

Mixing Directions

In blender combine all ingredients; blend until smooth.

Nutritional Facts

Makes 4 (1-cup) servings, each containing:

calories: 110
fat: 0.5 g
cholesterol: 1 mg
carbohydrate: 24 g
4% fat 87% carbohydrate 9% protein

protein: 2.5 g
sodium: 23 mg
fiber: 3 g
calcium: 68 mg

Tropical Smoothie

Ingredients

1 ripe medium banana, frozen and cut into pieces

8 ice cubes

1 cup chopped papaya

1/2 cup unsweetened pineapple juice

1/2 cup coconut milk

1 cup chopped mango

Mixing Directions

In blender combine all ingredients; blend until smooth.

Nutritional Facts

Makes 4 (1-cup) servings, each containing:

calories: 130
fat: 4.5 g
cholesterol: 0 mg
carbohydrate: 21.5 g
31% fat 66% carbohydrate 3% protein

protein: 1 g
sodium: 28 mg
fiber: 2 g
calcium: 19 mg

Kiwi Smoothie

Ingredients

4 ripe kiwis, peeled and cut into pieces
1/2 cup unsweetened pineapple juice
2 ripe medium bananas, frozen and cut into pieces
1/4 cup apple juice with vitamin C
8 ice cubes
1 tablespoon honey

Mixing Directions

In blender combine all ingredients, blend until smooth.

Nutritional Facts

Makes 4 (1-cup) servings, each containing:

calories: 140	protein: 1.5 g
fat: 0.5 g	sodium: 2 mg
cholesterol: 0 mg	fiber: 4 g
carbohydrate: 33 g	calcium: 29 mg

1.5% fat 94% carbohydrate 4.5% protein

Watermelon Smoothie

Ingredients

2 ripe kiwis, peeled and cut into pieces
4 ice cubes
2 cups chopped watermelon, seeds removed
3/4 cup apple juice with vitamin C
1 ripe medium banana, frozen and cut into pieces

Mixing Directions

In blender combine all ingredients; blend until smooth.

Nutrional Facts

Makes 4 (1-cup) servings, each containing:

calories: 97	protein: 1 g
fat: 0.5 g	sodium: 3 mg
cholesterol: 0 mg	fiber: 2 g
carbohydrate: 22.5 g	calcium: 21 mg

4% fat 92% carbohydrate 4% protein

Wildberry Cheesecake

Ingredients

Vegetable cooking spray

Crust:

1 1/2 cups graham cracker crumbs

1/4 cup apple juice with vitamin C

Filling:

2 tablespoons unflavored gelatin

1 package (8 oz.) lite cream cheese (Neufchatel)

1/2 cup water

1/4 cup sugar

2 cups 1% fat cottage cheese

1 tablespoon vanilla extract

1 cup nonfat ricotta cheese

1/2 cup Fruit Puree made with strawberries (see recipe)

Cooking Directions

For crust:

1. Preheat oven to 350° F.
2. Spray 9″ springform pan with cooking spray; set aside.
3. In medium bowl stir crumbs and apple juice until well combined.
4. With back of spoon press crumb mixture evenly into prepared pan.
5. Bake 5 minutes. Cool.

For filling:

1. In small saucepan sprinkle gelatin over water, let stand 5 minutes to soften.
2. Cook over low heat stirring, until dissolved. Set aside.
3. In food processor or blender process gelatin mixture and next 6 ingredients until smooth.
4. Stir in fruit puree.
5. Pour into prepared crust.
6. Refrigerate at least 2 hours or until set.

Nutritional Facts

Makes 10 servings, each containing:

calories: 180	protein: 12 g
fat: 2 g	sodium: 305 mg
cholesterol: 21 mg	fiber: 2 g
carbohydrate: 28 g	calcium: 116 mg

10% fat 63% carbohydrate 27% protein

Spa Anglaise

Ingredients

1/2 cup skim milk

1 teaspoon cornstarch or arrowroot

1/2 vanilla bean (about 4–5″ long), split lengthwise

1 cup plain nonfat yogurt

1 tablespoon light corn syrup

Cooking Directions

1. In small saucepan over high heat combine milk, vanilla bean, corn syrup, and cornstarch; bring to a boil, stirring.
2. Remove vanilla bean and scrape seeds back into milk mixture; discard bean.
3. Remove from heat: cool to room temperature. Stir in yogurt.
4. Refrigerate.

NOTE: To serve as a special dessert: On each of 8 dark colored dessert plates spread 3 T vanilla yogurt mixture. Place some Fruit Puree in small plastic bag: cut one bottom edge. Squeeze out dots of puree in circle around dish. With toothpick run through top center of dot to form heart.

Nutritional Facts

Makes 8 (3-T) servings, each containing:

calories: 30	protein: 2 g
fat: 0 g	sodium: 30 mg
cholesterol: 1 mg	fiber: 0 g
carbohydrate: 5 g	calcium: 75 mg

0% fat 70% carbohydrate 30% protein

Fruit Puree

Use this all-purpose puree as a sauce on ice cream, poached pears, crepes, waffles, pancakes . . . you name it!!

Ingredients

1 pound ripe fruit, peeled, pitted and cut in pieces, if needed (raspberries, strawberries, peaches, plums, figs, apricots, or cherries)

1/2 cup water

Mixing Directions

1. Place fruit and water in food processor or blender.
2. Puree for few seconds or at low speed until slightly chunky.
3. In small saucepan over medium-low heat simmer 5 minutes. Serve warm or cold.

Nutritional Facts

Makes 10 (1/4-cup) servings, each containing (per serving for raspberry):

calories: 22	protein: 0 g
fat: 0 g	sodium: 0 mg
cholesterol: 0 mg	fiber: 3.5 g
carbohydrate: 5 g	calcium: 10 mg

0% fat 100% carbohydrate 0% protein

TEN SINFUL DESSERTS FROM THE FOUR SEASONS RESORT AND CLUB AT LAS COLINAS IN IRVING, TEXAS—PASTRY CHEF RANDY GEHMAN

Cinnamon Yogurt Cheesecake with Raspberry Coulis

Ingredients

Cheesecake:

1 quart nonfat Yogurt Cheese (see recipe)

1 teaspoon vanilla

10 packages Nutrasweet (.35 oz. each)

2 tablespoons amaretto

1 prebaked graham-cracker shell (see recipe)

4 sheets gelatin

1 teaspoon cinnamon

2 egg whites

Raspberry Coulis:
1 pound frozen raspberries
juice of 1/2 lemon

Graham Cracker Shell:
4 ounces graham-cracker crumbs
1 tablespoon melted margarine
pinch of ginger
1 ounce honey

Cooking Directions

1. Reconstitute gelatin in ice water. When soft, melt slowly with the amaretto.
2. Mix the cheese, vanilla, and Nutrasweet until smooth.
3. Whip in the gelatin. Whip whites until soft peaks form, and fold into cheese mixture.
4. Place in prebaked shell, top with cinnamon, and swirl the top.
5. Refrigerate 2 hours.
6. Slice into 12 pieces and serve with Raspberry Coulis and sprig of mint.

To prepare graham-cracker shell: Blend ingredients. Press into a cake ring. Bake 5 minutes at 325° F.

To prepare raspberry coulis: Puree raspberries and juice; strain.

Makes 12 servings, each containing 176 calories.

Yogurt Cheese

Ingredients

2 quarts nonfat vanilla yogurt with artificial sweetener

Cooking Directions

Wrap nonfat yogurt in cheesecloth and drain for 24 hours.

Makes 1 quart, each 8 oz. serving contains approximately 200 calories

Fresh Strawberries with Chocolate Cream

Ingredients

Chocolate Cream:
1/2 cup skim ricotta
1 tablespoon Grand Marnier

1/2 cup skim milk
2 tablespoons cocoa
2 powdered egg whites (follow manufacturer's directions for amount of fluid needed to equal two egg whites)
2 ounces sugar
2 sheets gelatin

Cassis Puree:

6 ounces pureed cassis (blackberries)

1/4 cup water

2 packages Nutrasweet

1 ounce toasted almonds

Cooking Directions

1. Reconstitute gelatin in ice water. When soft, melt the gelatin with the Grand Marnier.
2. Mix the first 3 ingredients until smooth and beat the gelatin into this mixture.
3. Whip the powdered egg whites and sugar until a soft meringue forms and fold into above mixture.
4. Pour into 6 rings and chill for 2 hours.

To serve: Remove chocolate cream rings and place on a plate. Slice 2 large strawberries per plate. Discard ends and fan out into a circle around the chocolate creme. Place a bead of cassis coulise between each strawberry tip, and sprinkle chocolate cream with toasted almonds. Add mint leaf.

Makes 6 servings, each containing 299 calories.

Pumpkin Pie with Cranberry Coulis

Ingredients

Pumpkin Pie:

4 ounces Yogurt Cheese (see recipe)
13 ounces pumpkin puree
2 ounces nonfat milk powder
4 ounces water
1/2 teaspoon cinnamon
4 sheets gelatin
2 ounces water
2 egg whites
2 ounces sugar
1/4 teaspoon nutmeg

1/4 teaspoon cloves
1/8 teaspoon ginger
10 packages Nutrasweet

Cranberry Coulis:

12 ounces cranberries, chopped

zest of 1 orange

1 cinnamon stick and Nutrasweet to taste

Cooking Directions

1. Blend first 9 ingredients until smooth.
2. Soften gelatin sheets with water, melt, and add to above.
3. Whip egg whites and sugar into soft meringue, fold into above, and pour into prebaked pie shell (see Key Lime Pie recipe for Pie Shell).

To prepare coulis: Simmer all ingredients for 5 minutes. Cool.

Serve one slice pumpkin pie on plate with Cranberry Coulis on side.

Makes 12 servings, each containing 65 calories.

Pear-Blackberry Sorbet

Ingredients

10 medium baked pears

1 pint blackberries

3 ounces fructose

Cooking Directions

To prepare pear-blackberry puree: Puree baked pears with blackberries.

Puree fruit puree with fructose. Freeze in gelato machine (or ice-cream maker).

Serve 2 scoops in a chilled glass dessert bowl or frozen silver sorbetiere with mint garnish.

1 serving contains approximately 68 calories.

Sliced Oranges in Red Wine with Citrus Sorbet

Ingredients

12 large oranges

1 cup red wine

Citrus Sorbet:

1/4 cup lemon juice

3 ounces fructose

mint sprigs and candied orange zest for garnish

1 pint orange juice

Cooking Directions

1. Fillet oranges and marinate in wine for 3 to 4 hours.
2. Make sorbet by pureeing fruit juices with fructose.
3. Freeze in gelato machine (or ice-cream maker).

Alternative Method: If you do not have an ice cream maker you can freeze the citrus sorbet in a metal pan and stir hourly until the set up is grainy. You can put this mixture in a blender to smooth further. Return the mixture to the pan for freezing.

To serve: Arrange oranges in a pinwheel design on plate and top with Citrus Sorbet, mint, and candied orange zest.

Makes 8 servings, each containing approximately 171 calories.

Key Lime Pie with Blueberry Coulis

Ingredients

3 cups Yogurt Cheese (see recipe)

1/3 cup lime juice

6 packages Nutrasweet

3 sheets gelatin

2 tablespoons tequila

2 powdered egg whites (Follow manufacturer's directions for amount of fluid needed to equal two egg whites.)

Pie Shell:

4 oz. graham-cracker crumbs

pinch of ginger

1 tablespoon margarine, melted

1 ounce honey

Blueberry Coulis:

2 ounces sugar

2 ounces fructose

10 ounces frozen blueberries

Cooking Directions

1. Blend Yogurt Cheese, lime juice, and Nutrasweet.
2. Soften gelatin and melt with tequila. Add to above.
3. Whip powdered egg whites and sugar until soft peaks form. Add to above and place in prebaked shell.
4. Refrigerate 2 hours.

To serve: Place one slice on a plate with Blueberry Coulis. Garnish with mint and lightly candied lime zest.

Pie shell: Blend ingredients. Press into 10″ pie tin and bake 5 minutes at 350° F.

Blueberry Coulis: Thaw frozen blueberries and blend with fructose in food processor.

Makes 10 servings each containing approximately 179 calories

Sautéed Bananas with Honey and Vanilla Ice Milk

Ingredients

1/4 cup apple juice, unsweetened

Pinch cinnamon

Pinch ginger

1/2 medium banana, sliced on long bias

Pinch cornstarch

1 tablespoon honey

Vanilla ice milk

coconut flakes

mint sprigs

Cooking Directions

1. Cook apple juice, spices, and honey to a sauce.
2. Simmer sliced banana for 1 minute in above sauce.

To serve: Arrange bananas in a soup bowl and tip with a medium scoop of vanilla ice milk. Garnish with a few toasted coconut flakes and mint.

Makes 1 serving containing approximately 257 calories.

Peach Sorbet/Mango Sorbet

Ingredients

1 quart peach puree (see fruit puree recipe)

1 quart mango puree (see fruit puree recipe)

3 ounces fructose

1 quart water

Cooking Directions

1. Blend fruit puree, fructose, and water.
2. Freeze in a gelato machine (or ice cream maker).

Alternate Method: Freeze in a metal pan and stir hourly until the set up is grainy. You can put this mixture in an electric blender to smooth further. Return the mixture to the metal pan for freezing.

Serve in a chilled glass dessert bowl or frozen silver sorbetiere, 2 scoops with mint garnish.

Makes 16 servings, each containing approximately 59 calories.

Baked Pear with Blackberries, Cassis Yogurt

Ingredients

1 D'Anjou pear

2 ounces blackberries

1 teaspoon lemon juice

Cassis Yogurt:

1/4 cup lowfat yogurt

2 tablespoons blackberry pear juice

1 tablespoon Cassis Liqueur

Cooking Directions

1. Peel and core pear. Slice in half lengthwise.
2. Bake in oven at 350° for 25 minutes with blackberries and lemon juice.
3. Baste pears every 5 minutes and bake al denté.
4. Brush pear with syrup prior to slicing.

To serve: Fan pear lengthwise, making sure not to cut through at the neck end. Place the yogurt sauce on the plate and place the pear on top. Sprinkle yogurt with chopped pistachios and garnish with a few raspberries.

Makes 2 servings, each containing approximately 116 calories.

SUM IT UP!

Plenty of water and fiber, a balanced collection of vitamin- and mineral-rich foods, antioxidant-rich diet. What do they have in common? These valuable components contribute not only to the health of your body but ultimately to your skin's health. Taking care of your skin is more than just applying creme to your skin. Smart skin care is actually a twofold regimen: internal and external. Applying sunscreens, avoiding the sun, and applying the correct skin care products is the external aspect of skin care. Good nutrition is the internal form because what you consume daily (if it is well balanced and you drink plenty of water) will help nourish and hydrate your skin. If you have any doubts about the quality of your diet, refer to the power food chart and nutrient-rich food chart to give you ideas on how to change any bad habits you may have. And if you're bored with your meals, try the exciting collection of spa recipes that have been selected for your skin needs. It is time you thought more about what you eat each day because it can truly make a difference in your life. If you're not sure how to begin, use the nutritional advice, informational facts, and delicious spa recipes in this chapter; they will help guide you on a path to quality eating.

C H A P T E R

Five

TURN YOUR HOME INTO A SPA FOR THE WEEKEND

Does your schedule resemble a hurried, fast-paced treadmill that makes it difficult for you to take a breath? Do you feel frazzled, drained, and stressed-out? Do you desperately feel that you need to get away? Well, despair no more! You've just been invited to a pampering two-day escape. You say you can't get away? Well, I'm going to show you how to transform your home into an exclusive beauty retreat for two days. You will learn the art of escaping without even leaving your neighborhood. There are no excuses to deprive and neglect yourself anymore.

This at-home spa program will be like having your very own staff of beauty experts—a nutritionist, facialist, body therapist, masseuse, and personal trainer. A specially designed and structured repertoire of exotic facial and body beauty treatments, delicious foods, and plenty of relaxation time awaits you on any weekend you choose. The purpose of the at-home spa concept is to teach you how to slow up a busy schedule and be good to yourself. You will discover how to pamper your body from head to toe and renew your spirits.

This at-home spa weekend does not do away with the need to visit a destination spa, day spa, or esthetician. It's also a wonderful experience to be treated by a skin expert and spa specialist too. See Chapter 13 for more details.

For now, come join me in an experience you will never forget.

YOUR PRESCRIPTION FOR BECOMING STRESS-FREE

A weekend of pampering can renew your spirits and revive your looks. This weekend will offer a collection of healthful regimens; each is explained in detail to help keep your weekend organized and running smoothly. You will find exclusive recipes from famous spas, luxurious pampering treatments, relaxation advice, and sensible fitness techniques.

Your one evening and two days of total indulgence have been mapped out with a complete timetable to help you keep your at-home spa routine on schedule. All your supply needs and preparation work have also been listed.

One of the most important bits of advice I can give you to help you maximize the therapeutic value of your at-home spa weekend is to have everything prepared in advance so when the weekend arrives you can feel like a guest in your own home.

Nutrition—Meals That Will Beautify Your Skin

This will be a weekend of sinfully good foods and desserts that are actually nutritious. You will enjoy breakfasts, lunches, dinners, desserts, and snacks that are exclusive to famous spas. These simple yet healthy recipes take very little time to prepare, and many of them can be made a day or two in advance. If you choose not to cook for the weekend you can treat yourself to dinner at a neighborhood restaurant. Eat in or take the meal home—the option is yours. But remember when selecting from the menu try to choose a meal that is light and healthful so it will follow the theme of your at-home spa weekend.

Pampering Beauty Treatments from Head to Toe That Will Boost Your Self-Esteem

It is time that you treated yourself like royalty. A little pampering goes a long way. This weekend you will be buffed, polished, deep cleansed, moisturized, and wrapped. Each exotic treatment is designed to enhance your skin's beauty potential. You will feel like a new person.

Water Relaxation Techniques

Discover how your bath and shower can become your best friends. You will indulge in one of the most ancient forms of pampering and relaxation—water therapy. Escape from stress as you soak in waters that have been treated with natural plant and fruit essences or minerals salts.

Music Enlightenment That Will Help You Lift Your Spirits

The sounds of the ocean, and the forest, wind, birds, and brooks, as well as new age instrumentals should always be played in the background. This is called white noise, and it will gently blanket any outside noise that may surround you. This type of music should be wafting though each of your special rooms. If you do not have this type of music selection go to your nearest music store and ask a salesperson to direct you. This type of music has become very popular due to its soothing therapeutic effect on the spirit.

Relaxing Massage

Massage is the perfect antidote to stress. When you feel relaxed you look and feel refreshed. This weekend you will enjoy massage treatments that include self-massage, an aromatherapy shower and rubdown, salt and oil rub, and a soothing aromatherapy scalp massage. These are just a few treatments that are part of your beauty regimen for the weekend. To make your at-home spa weekend even more exciting you could treat yourself to a professional massage. The cost for a massage is approximately $30 to $40 for a half hour and $50 to $60 for an hour. You can either go to a day spa in your area or have a certified massage therapist come to your home for the half hour or full hour massage. A good massage is worth every penny.

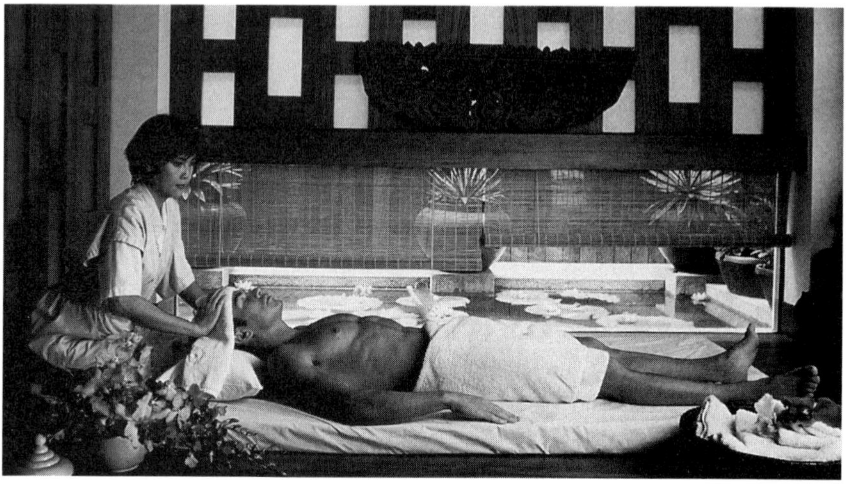

The Oriental Spa, Thai Health and Beauty Center in Bangkok, Thailand. This exceptional "Oriental Spa Massage" technique was created exclusively for the Oriental Spa. It combines Thai Massage with the traditional Oriental deep tissue massage technique.

Read Self-Help Books

Now is the time to catch up on some reading and learn something new. Learn more about beauty, food, cooking, fitness, health, meditation, and so forth. Accomplishing this task is good for one's spirit.

CREATING A SPA ENVIRONMENT

Setting the stage is as important as the actual beauty treatments. Exclusive spas go to great lengths to create the perfect environment to help you achieve total relaxation. Visual beauty, scent, sound, and lighting are all gently melded to become an important part of your spa experience.

To make your two-day stay at home a truly relaxing and pampering experience, you will want to transform your environment, room by room, to give it the ambiance of a luxurious beauty retreat. You don't have to change your whole living space. Just select four areas that will be important focal points for your pampered weekend: your dining area, your bathroom, your bedroom, and one quiet corner somewhere in your living quarters. Here are some suggested ways to utilize your space to its best advantage.

Dining area—spa meals, snacks, and herbal tea breaks

Bathroom—water relaxation remedies, facials, and body treatments

Bedroom—mini essential oil relaxation breaks, body wrap, manicures and pedicures, quiet reading time and meditation

Quiee corner—music enlightenment, reading, sipping herbal tea and healthy fruit juices

Beautify Your Surroundings

Luxurious spas have fresh-cut flowers in every room. Make sure you have flowers in view. Where should you place your flowers? Your dining area, foyer, bathroom, bedroom, and your quiet corner should be adorned with fragrant blossoms. If you don't have enough vases, borrow a few from your friends or go to a party-supply store. I'm sure you will find small vases for under $2. If you are on a budget, purchase your flowers at your local supermarket. Bunches of flowers range from $3.99 to $5.99. You can pick up two or three bouquets and divide them among four or five small vases.

Now, let's talk about your dining area. How are you going to feel like a guest in your own home without spending too much money? Go to your nearest discount department store or import outlet. Purchase two pretty place mats and several cloth napkins. Select the kind you imagine yourself eating off in a spa. The cost of these items is nominal; you should spend no more than $2 to $3 per place mat or napkin. Then I want you to promise me something. Every time you have your very special spa meals during the weekend set your table as if you were expecting company. Take out your Sunday-best dishes and glassware. Fold your napkin and place it either on your plate or in your water goblet. Have a tray handy in case you want to indulge yourself and have breakfast or your delicious herbal tea break in bed. And don't forget to use a very special cup and saucer for your herbal tea.

Lighting and Aroma

Keep your lights low. A dimly lit environment can soothe frazzled nerves. In the evening you can light your new spa quarters with candles. This is a very important part of the experience because there is something extremely mesmerizing and calming about a flickering flame. Double the benefits of the candle therapy by making them scented. The aroma will fill the air of your pampering palace to help you set the mood of luxury. The cost of the candles is quite low. You can find small scented candles for approximately 60 cents, and they will burn for about six hours. Glass holders for the candles will cost a little under a dollar. Each of your special rooms should have at least three candles.

CALENDAR OF EVENTS

Your weekend of pampering begins on Friday evening. It's time to unwind from the events of the week and enjoy yourself. A week before your special weekend begins review the calendar of events and the preparation section.

Friday Evening

5:00 to 5:30 P.M.	Evening stroll
5:30 to 7:00 P.M.	Spa dinner
7:00 to 8:30 P.M.	Herbal and citrus spa pedicure
8:30 to 9:00 P.M.	Dry Brushing and Soothing Night Time Essential Oil Soak
9:00 to 10:00 P.M.	Quiet time

Saturday

7:00 to 7:30 A.M.	Quiet time
7:30 to 8:30 A.M.	Spa breakfast
8:30 to 9:30 A.M.	Morning stroll
9:30 to 10:30 A.M.	Pore cleansing aromatherapy compress-conditioning wheat-germ facial and décolleté treatment
10:30 to 11:30 A.M.	Exercise of your choice

11.30 to 11:45 A.M.	Snack: Tropical Smoothie
11:45 to 1:00 P.M.	Aromatherapy shower and rubdown
1:00 to 2:00 P.M.	Spa lunch
2:00 to 3:00 P.M.	Meditation
3:00 to 5:00 P.M.	Escape for two hours
5:00 to 7:00 P.M.	Spa dinner
7:00 to 9: 00 P.M.	Salt and oil rub and essential oil soak
9:00 to 10:00 P.M.	Quiet time

Sunday

7:00 to 7:30 A.M.	Quiet time
7:30 to 8:30 A.M.	Spa breakfast
8:30 to 9:30 A.M.	Morning stroll
9:30 to 10:30 A.M.	Exercise of your choice
10:30 to 10:45 A.M.	Snack: Kiwi Smoothie
10:45 to 11:45 A.M.	Essential oil hair and scalp treatment
11:45 to 1:00 P.M.	Gentle face, throat and décolleté skin polishing
1:00 to 2:00 P.M.	Spa lunch
2:00 to 3:00 P.M.	Rose water spa manicure
3:00 to 5:00 P.M.	Escape for two hours
5:00 to 7:00 P.M.	Spa dinner
7:00 to 9:00 P.M.	Mud body masque/wrap and warm herbal soak and cool shower
9:00 to 10:00 P.M.	Quiet time

Preparation Is the Key

How to Dodge Your Responsibilities for the Weekend You won't be able to enjoy your weekend if you have a schedule of errands to do for either yourself or for your family. If you are going to successfully pull off this weekend you will need to do all your chores in advance. Remember you have to completely clear your calendar from your day-to-day responsibilities. The only thing I want you to focus on is yourself. Now doesn't that sound great? Here are some preparation tips:

1. If you have small children find a responsible babysitter. This weekend can be made special for your children also by planning exciting activities or outings with the babysitter. The children should sleep at the babysitter's house. You can also ask a family member for help.
2. Laundry, house cleaning, food shopping, and any other errands should be completed before the weekend. Try to accomplish them by Wednesday or Thursday evening. Don't leave the chores for Friday; I don't want you to have a nervous breakdown trying to get ready for this weekend. Get all the drudgeries out of the way. I want you to feel as if you're getting ready for a holiday.

Spa Weekend Shopping List To help you organize your spa weekend I have listed the supplies you will need and where to find them. Many of these items you may have at home. I've also tried to suggest alternative items to help you keep your costs down.

Supplies from the Supermarket: If you decide to cook for yourself on your spa weekend, be sure to read over all the wonderful recipes in Chapter 4 before you start your weekend. Make a list of the items you'll need from the store and do your shopping in advance. Even if you're not planning to cook, be sure to get the following items for your beauty treatments:

- Chamomile tea, rosehip tea
- Fresh rosemary, sage, parsley, peppermint leaves
- Fresh lime
- Small piece of cheesecloth

Environment Enhancers: These supplies can be found in discount stores, import outlets, and department stores.

- Flowers (supermarkets have economically priced bouquets)
- Scented and nonscented candles
- Decorative place mats and cloth napkins

Beauty Supplies and Face, Body, and Bath Accessories: These supplies can be found in many salons, bath shops, and drug stores.

- Olive oil-based soap for cleansing the body
- Plastic shower cap
- White cotton gloves
- Natural-bristle complexion cleansing brush. This brush is designed with natural boars' bristles to produce a gentle exfoliating and massaging action, as it effectively removes surface impurities, dirt, and makeup. This brush should be used with your cleansing creme. Please note that if you have acne skin you should not use this brush.
- Natural-bristle body brush. Try to locate either a 10-inch-handle brush or a 16-inch-wooden-handle brush with a detachable brush. A bath brush is a perfect tool for a balanced body-care regimen. It offers just the right amount of stimulation and exfoliation.
- Sea-wool bathing sponge. This is used for cleansing the body in the shower or bath. The size of this item is approximately 4 to 6 inches. The strong wool sea sponge is coarse in texture but is exceptionally soft and durable.

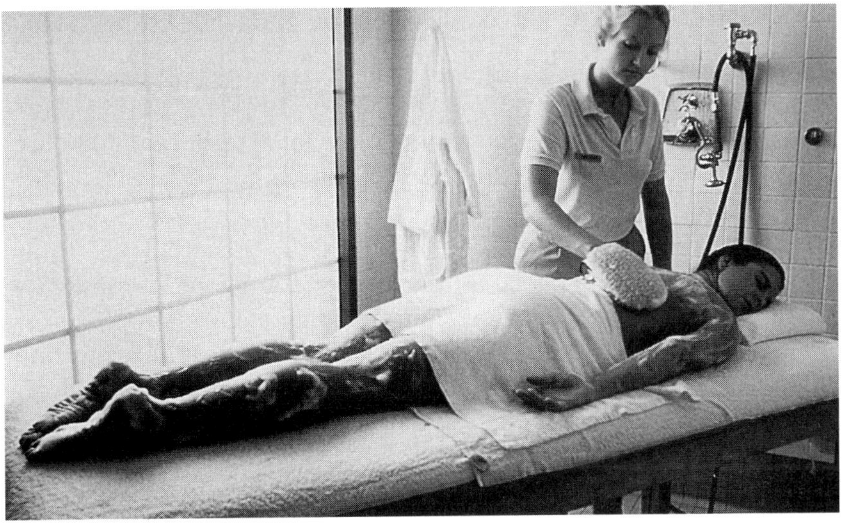

The Spa at the Four Seasons Resort and Club at Las Colinas, Texas. A delightful full body exfoliating treatment designed to make the skin feel as smooth as silk.

- Foot basin for spa pedicure
- Pumice stone and stick
- Cuticle nipper, medium-grade file, fine-grade file, and smooth nail buffer
- Inflatable pillow for baths

Supplies from Your Home:

- Large bath towels
- Robe
- Small kitchen bowl for manicure
- Small plastic container to hold coarse salt
- Old sheet
- Warm thermal blanket
- Two cups coarse salt
- Disposable cups
- Base coat, nail polish, and top coat
- Shampoo
- Conditioner
- Nonacetone nail polish remover
- Your skin-care products: cleanser, toner, day moisturizer, facial scrub, night creme, unscented body lotion
- Unused plastic drop cloth for mud treatment
- String and a 6″ x 6″ piece of cheesecloth for herbal and citrus pedicure

Supplies of Essential Oils and Body Oils Essential oils (found in many salons and specialty bath shops) should be purchased in small bottles because they are extremely concentrated. Store in a cool, dry place and keep out of direct sunlight. Base oils and body oils are purchased in larger sizes because they are mixed with the essential oils and massaged all over the body.

- Chamomile oil
- Peppermint oil
- Lavender oil

- Eucalyptus oil
- Rose oil
- Orange-blossom oil*
- Lemon oil*
- Rosemary oil*
- Thyme oil*
- Juniper oil*
- Base and body oils: Pure squalane oil, almond oil, macadamia oil, and jojoba oil. If you want to keep expenses down you can select one of these oils.

*These oils can be substituted with preblended oils that are formulated to be calming or stimulating. Take your pick.

Supplies from the Health Store

- Wheat-germ oil
- Royal gelee powder
- Aloe vera gel
- Cocoa butter

Steps to Take Before Your Spa Weekend Begins

Organize all the supplies you will need for each of the treatments and your menu. This will eliminate the stress of not finding what you need. You may want to prepare a slip of paper for each of the treatments so you can list what you will need.

THE SPA PROGRAM

Friday Evening

5:00 to 5:30 P.M. *Evening stroll.* Unwind from the events of the day with a leisurely stroll. Meditate on pleasant thoughts. This walk will help whet your appetite for dinner.

5:30 to 7:00 P.M. *Spa dinner.* Try the delicious Grilled Honey Basil Chicken with Twice-Baked Potatoes, compliments of sports and spa nutritionist Cheryl Hartsough, RD, LD, of the PGA National Spa, Palm Beach Gardens, Florida. Turn to Chapter Four for complete recipe instructions.

7:00 to 8:30 P.M. *Herbal and citrus spa pedicure.* Take your tired feet and soak them in delightful, cleansing waters. This herbal and citrus footbath will cleanse as well as refresh your feet. Learn how to treat your feet like royalty with this pampering spa pedicure.

Supplies

- Large foot basin
- Two bath towels (one towel is to be placed under the pedicure basin and the other is to be placed on your lap to protect your clothing and to dry your feet)
- Pumice stone and pumice stick
- Natural-bristle body brush or abrasive mitt (both can be found in many salons, department stores, and bath shops). An alternative product you can use if you can't find either of these items is a natural-bristle nail brush.
- Herb and citrus fruit: 2 teaspoons sage, 3 teaspoons parsley, 1 teaspoon rosemary, 8 peppermint leaves, 1/2 lime
- One 6″ x 6″ square piece of cheesecloth and a piece of string
- Sweet almond oil and cocoa butter
- Toenail clipper, file, and nail buffer (very smooth file)
- Base coat, nail polish, top coat
- Unscented body lotion
- Optional peppermint or eucalyptus oil

Step One: Preparation. Prepare your herbal and citrus packet by placing all the herbs and half a lime into the cheesecloth. Then tie the cloth closed with the string and place it into the large foot basin and fill with hot water. Let the herbs and lime steep for five minutes. While herbs and lime are steeping lay out all your supplies.

Step Two: Soak and nail shaping. Soak feet for 10 minutes in the herbal and citrus water. Then clip your toenails and smooth and shape your nails with the file. After your toenails are shaped, apply a few drops of sweet almond oil to the cocoa butter and massage on each toenail and then the entire foot and ankle. Place both feet back into the foot bath for another five minutes.

Step Three: Exfoliate. While your feet are still in the foot basin take your natural-bristle brush, abrasive mitt, or natural-bristle nail brush and vigorously massage your feet until they tingle. Then remove feet from the water and gently buff the soles and any calluses with the pumice stone. This will help to remove dead skin. Next take your pumice stick and push back the cuticle on each toenail. Dab a drop of sweet almond oil on each of your toenails and smooth any ridges or flakiness with the smooth buffer. To use the buffer properly, buff in one direction with no more than 10 strokes. Dip your feet in the foot bath, then towel dry.

Step Four: Conditioning. Massage both feet with sweet almond oil. (Add two drops of peppermint oil or eucalyptus to a portion of almond oil if you want a cooling sensation.) When massaging your feet use a strong kneading type of movement. Use both hands and exert pressure: Begin with the toe, concentrate on each joint, then the balls of the feet, the arch, the heel, the ankle, and the back of your legs. Wipe off each toenail to remove oil before polishing your nails. Apply basecoat, two coats of polish, and a top coat.

Step Five: Unwind. Relax for 20 minutes with your feet elevated and sip a cup of your favorite herbal tea.

8:30 to 9:15 P.M. *Dry Brushing and Soothing Nighttime Essential Oil Soak.* Slowly slip into a fragrant bath of herbal, floral, and citrus oils to help you escape from the stress of the day. Close your eyes and imagine you are in some exotic spa and you are being pampered. Breathe in the natural essences, feel the warm soothing water on your skin, and gain peace of mind. This bath is just a delicious prelude to your spa weekend at home.

Supplies

- Robe
- 3 drops chamomile oil, 2 drops peppermint oil, 6 drops lavender, 3 drops orange oil (Alternate product: All of these essen-

tial oils can be substituted by one "soothing" premixed blend of essential oils. Always follow manufacturer's directions.)

- Natural-bristle body brush
- Inflatable bath pillow
- Large natural sea-wool bathing sponge
- Unscented body oil or pure squalane oil (derived from olives)
- Olive-oil-based bath soap for cleansing the body

Step One: Preparation. Play soft music and light a candle; place it near the tub. Then add 3 drops chamomile, 3 drops peppermint, 6 drops lavender, and 3 drops orange blossom essential oil into running bath water.

Step Two: Dry brushing. Gently massage your skin while it is still dry with a natural-bristle body brush, utilizing short strokes. Begin with your feet, work up the thighs, buttocks, torso, and arms. Then add 1 drop of chamomile oil and 1 drop lavender oil to a portion of unscented body oil or pure squalane oil. Massage onto your skin while it is dry. Be generous with the oil and concentrate on problem areas that are prone to flaky skin and calluses (knees, elbows, and backs of arms).

Step Three: Conditioning. Once you have drenched your body with the soothing, skin-softening oil, step into the essential-oil-enriched water. Relax and soak for 20 minutes. Close your eyes and enjoy the scents of the natural essences.

Step Four: Cleansing. Take your natural sea-wool sponge and olive-oil-based soap and cleanse your skin.

Step Five: Calming. Wrap yourself in a large, thick terry towel and pat dry. Add a drop of chamomile oil and a drop of lavender to your unscented body lotion. Massage into your skin. Slip into comfortable bed clothes.

9:15 to 10:00 P.M. *Evening Quiet Time.* Relax, put your feet up, and treat yourself to a cup of your favorite herbal tea. This is a perfect time to collect your thoughts and prepare yourself for a peaceful night's sleep. Quality sleep is a very important part of skin care, because as you rest your skin has a chance to renew itself.

Saturday

***7:00 to 7:30* A.M.** *Morning Quiet Time.* Don't jump out of bed this morning! Remember you have no chores to do. The only thing on your agenda is a day of pampering. Before you get out of bed listen to some soothing music and indulge in a nice long stretch. Next drink a tall glass (at least 10 ounces) of either cranberry water or apple water to start your day. (Mixing directions: 2 ounces of juice to 8 ounces of water.)

***7:30 to 8:30* A.M.** *Spa Breakfast.* Never skip breakfast, because it is the fuel for your motor. If you have plenty of energy it will help you look refreshed and youthful. Light and nourishing is the theme for today's spa breakfast. One cup of fresh nonfat plain yogurt (110 calories, 0 fat) with a half cup of fresh or frozen blueberries, strawberries, or kiwis (40 calories, 0 fat).

***8:30 to 9:30* A.M.** *Morning Power Walk.* Walking is probably the safest form of cardiovascular exercise because you can do it at your own pace. How can walking help your skin? Any time you improve your circulation you bring an abundent blood supply to your skin. This increased blood supply nourishes your skin and helps to keep it functioning properly.

A few tips on walking: Start slowly with a warm-up for at least 10 to 15 minutes. Then increase your speed slightly for 15 minutes to 30 minutes. Then slow down your pace for the last 15 minutes. You should wear layered clothes so you can peel off a layer or two as you warm up. When you complete your walk, have a tall 10-ounce glass of cranberry water.

***9:30 to 10:30* A.M.** *Pore Cleansing Aromatherapy Compress.* Wrap your face in a warm, moist towel that has been saturated with a blend of deep-pore cleansing herbal and floral essences. Deep cleansing sprigs of rosemary, soothing and healing chamomile, and vitamin C-rich rosehips steep into a unique fluid that will help cleanse dirt and makeup from your pores. This compress therapy is also extremely soothing to your skin and spirits.

Supplies

- Kitchen bowl
- Hand towel (approximately 15″ x 24″) (Use an old towel because this treatment will stain the towel.)
- 2 sprigs fresh rosemary
- 2 chamomile tea bags
- 1 rosehip tea bag
- 1 cup boiling water
- 2 cups warm water

Step One: Preparation. Add the 2 sprigs of rosemary, 2 chamomile tea bags, and 1 rosehip tea bag to one cup of boiling water in the kitchen bowl and let it steep for 10 minutes. Then remove the herbs and tea bags from the bowl and add the 2 cups warm water.

Immerse towel in the bowl until it is completely saturated with the herbal solution. Then lift towel over the bowl and wring out excess moisture. Save the balance of the herbal water in the bowl.

Step Two: Deep cleansing. Your face should be completely cleansed and free of all makeup. While you're in a reclining position wrap the towel around your face leaving your nose exposed. Keep the compress on for 10 to 15 minutes. This treatment is the perfect prelude to your Conditioning Wheat Germ Facial.

Conditioning Wheat Germ Facial and Décolleté Treatment. Replenish your skin with the vitamin E wheat-germ oil, protein-rich royal gelee powder, and healing aloe vera gel. This treatment marries three natural ingredients with exceptional conditioning properties. This is the perfect restorative remedy for neglected skin. (Please note if you have acne skin and are under medical care do not do this treatment.)

Supplies

- Natural-bristle complexion brush
- Cleanser

- Royal gelee powder (You can locate this item in most health-food stores.)
- Aloe vera gel (You can locate this item in most health-food stores and drug stores.)
- Wheat-germ oil (You can locate this item in most herbal stores, bath shops, and health-food stores.)
- Day moisturizer

Step One: Preparation. Mix 1 teaspoonful of royal gelee powder, 1 teaspoonful of wheat-germ oil with 3 ounces of aloe vera gel.

Step Two: Cleansing and exfoliating. Pull your hair back in a headband or turban. Splash warm water on your face and then apply the cleanser to your décolleté, throat, and face. Gently massage entire area with the complexion brush over the cleanser in a circular movement beginning at the base of the décolleté and working your way upward. Rinse with water.

Step Three: Conditioning. Apply the skin-conditioning wheat-germ masque you've prepared and massage a portion of it on your décolleté, throat, and face. Then apply a second application of masque over the first. Relax by lying down for 15 to 20 minutes. Rinse well with the warm rosemary, chamomile, and rosehip solution you have saved from the compress treatment. Apply your moisturizer.

***10:30 to 11:30* A.M.** *Exercise of your choice.* Improve the quality of your skin by improving the overall heath of your body with exercise. Walking, jogging, running, aerobics, yoga, calisthenics, ice skating, roller skating, biking, golf, tennis, badminton are just a few ways in which you can be on the move. Select a sport or exercise that interests you and have fun. (Before starting any exercise program always consult with your physician.)

***11:30 to 11:45* A.M.** *Spa Snack.* Time for a low-calorie and refreshing mango-papaya snack. Try the delicious Tropical Smoothie Drink, compliments of Cheryl Hartsough, RD, LD, sports and spa nutritionist for the PGA National Spa, Palm Beach Gardens, Florida. See Chapter Four for recipe instructions.

11:45 to 1:00 P.M. *Customized Aromatherapy Shower and Essential Oil Rubdown.* Jump into your shower and improve your mood as you mingle with the floral, herbal, and citrus essential oils. Select the essential oil formula that is right for the moment.

Essential Oil Formulas

RELAXING: 2 drops orange blossom, 2 drops chamomile

STIMULATING: 4 drops peppermint, 2 drops rosemary, 1 drop eucalyptus

REFRESHING: 4 drops lemon, 2 drops peppermint

Mixing Directions:

Mix your selected formula into 3 ounces of unscented body oil in a disposable plastic cup or plastic travel-size bottle with nozzle. If you want to keep your expenses down you can substitute these oils with a premixed relaxing, stimulating, or refreshing blend. Follow manufacturers directions.

Step One: Conditioning. Jump into a warm to hot shower for 1 minute, then massage a small portion of essential oil mixture all over your body. Shower for another 2 to 3 minutes. Turn water off and while still in the shower stall or tub pat yourself dry. Massage your selected essential oil mixture all over your body. Pay particular attention to your ankles, knees, wrists, and throat. Slip into a comfortable robe and relax for 10 minutes with your feet elevated. Don't shower for a few hours because you don't want to wash off the benefits of the essential oil.

1:00 to 2:00 P.M. *Spa Lunch.* Enjoy this power lunch that was designed by Cheryl Hartsough, LD, RD., sports and spa nutritionist for the PGA National Resort Spa, Palm Beach Gardens, Florida. Rich in vitamins and minerals the Butternut Squash Soup (68 calories) and Hot Spinach Salad (160 calories) offers a nourishing yet light lunch. See Chapter Four for complete recipe instructions.

2:00 to 3:00 P.M. *Quiet Time.* Relax and meditate for an hour and renew your inner self. If you are not sure how to meditate there are quite a few books on the subject and this may be the perfect time to learn something new. Try an essential oil break. Mix 1

cup warm water with 3 drops of lavender. Moisten 3 cotton pads and wring out excess moisture. Place pads on forehead and wrists (pulse points) and relax for 5 minutes.

3:00 to 5:00 P.M. *Escape for two hours.* Disconnecting from your schedule for a couple of hours works wonders. Unrestricted recreation can be fun because it can be like an adventure. What should you do for your two hours? You probably have a long list of fun things you want to do but never get to because you don't have the time—well, now's the time. Go to the movies or rent a movie, catch up on reading, go to a museum, stroll and go window shopping, sit in the park, or just take a nap. These are just a few things you can do during your escape but remember whatever you do should be stress-free.

5:00 to 7:00 P.M. *Spa Dinner.* It's dinner time and I'm sure you're hungry. Sports and spa nutritionist Cheryl Hartsough, RD, LD, from the PGA National Resort Spa, Palm Beach Gardens, Florida, has created a southwestern dish that is low in fat and high in flavor. Long Horn Gazpacho (65 calories, 0 fat) Smoked Turkey Quesadilla (345 calories, 9 grams of fat). See Chapter Four for complete recipes instructions.

7:00 to 9:00 P.M. *Salt and Warm Oil Rub with an Essential Oil Soak.* After this treatment, your skin will feel as silky and smooth as baby skin. The salt will slough away any traces of rough flaky skin. This invigorating beauty remedy will make you feel like a new person.

Supplies

- Coarse sea salt
- Almond oil
- Chamomile, eucalyptus, thyme, lavender, peppermint essential oils
- Large bath towel
- Unscented body lotion

Step One: Preparation. Fill tub with warm water and add 2 drops of chamomile, 2 drops thyme, 6 drops of lavender, 3 drops of peppermint essential oil. Fill a plastic container with the coarse salt and place it next to the tub.

Step Two: Exfoliation. Soak for one minute in the tub to moisten skin. Then sit at the edge of the tub and massage the sweet almond oil all over your body. Then take a handful of coarse salt and begin the exfoliating process, start with your feet and work your way up to the thighs, the buttocks, abdomen, torso, arms, shoulders, and décolleté. When massaging your skin use a little extra pressure with the salt and oil on areas that have calluses such as soles of feet, knees, elbows. Your massage movements should be slow, circular motions. Once you have completed the sloughing treatment just slip into the essential oil enriched waters and soak for 20 minutes. Enjoy the fragrance from the natural essences and relax.

Step Three: Conditioning. Step out of the bath and pat yourself dry. Then add 1 drop of peppermint and 1 drop of eucalyptus essential oils to a portion (approximately 1 ounce) of your unscented body lotion. Rub the lotion into your skin with an invigorating circular massage movement. Then slip into comfortable lounging or bed clothes.

9:00 to 10:00 P.M. *Quiet Time.* Curl up in your most comfortable chair or sofa with a cup of your favorite herbal tea or naturally flavored fruit water. Read a book or reflect on the events of the day. Enjoy your hour of peacefulness.

10:00 P.M. *Time to go to bed.* A good night's sleep is a very important part of caring for your skin. Sleeping tips: Wear comfortable sleeping attire. If your surrounding area is noisy, buy yourself a pair of ear plugs or play soft background music.

Sunday

7:00 to 7:30 A.M. *Morning Quiet Time.* Don't jump right out of bed when you wake. To start your day on the right foot gently wake your body. While still in bed think about all the wonderful things you are going to experience today. Then gently stretch by starting with your feet and working upward. Then fluff your pillow up behind you so you can sit up for a few moments. Cleanse yourself internally by drinking a large glass of plain water or cranberry water (mix 2 ounces cranberry juice with 8 ounces water).

***7:30 to 8:30* A.M.** *Spa Breakfast.* A hearty, low-fat breakfast is a great way to start your day. Mix 1 cup oatmeal with 1 teaspoon raisins and a dash of cinnamon (165 calories), 1/2 cup skim milk (45 calories), 1/2 cup unsweetened applesauce (50 calories).

***8:30 to 9:30* A.M.** *Morning Power Walk.* Walking is great for your skin because it improves your circulation and it helps to relieve stress—and we know what a negative effect stress has on the skin. Exercise produces a hormone called endorphin, which gives you a calm feeling. Before you begin to walk it is always a good idea to stretch your muscles and to warm up slowly. Walk slowly for the first and last 10 minutes. Don't forget to wear layered clothing so you won't overheat.

***9:30 to 10:30* A.M.** *Exercise of your choice.* Extend your morning walk or do aerobics, calisthenics, or yoga—the choice is yours. Wear comfortable clothing and proper footwear. (If you have not exercised in a while always consult with your physician first.)

***10:30 to 10:45* A.M.** *Spa Snack: Kiwi Smoothie.* This treat tastes too good to be true, and it's fat-free and low in calories. Cheryl Hartsough, LD, RD, nutritionist for the PGA National Resort Spa, Palm Beach Gardens, Florida, suggests that you drink the Kiwi Smoothie as a refreshing morning treat to help curb your appetite. See Chapter Four for recipe.

***10:45 to 11:00* A.M.** *Soothing Aromatherapy Scalp Massage.* Release tension and stress as well as condition your scalp with the natural essences of chamomile and lavender.

Supplies

- 4 drops lavender essential oil
- 2 drops chamomile essential oil
- 1 ounce squalane oil (derived from olives)

Step One: Preparation. Mix 4 drops lavender oil, 2 drops of chamomile oil into 1 ounce of pure squalane oil.

Step Two: Soothing and conditioning. Dip the fingertips of both hands into the essential oil mixture. Then place your fingertips at the beginning of your hairline at the forehead and temples. Proceed massaging with small circular movements and moderate pressure. Always concentrate your thoughts on the area you are massaging. Work your way back to the nape of your neck and repeat this movement until the entire scalp has been massaged. Do not rinse because this treatment is a prelude to the Jojoba Hair and Scalp Conditioning Facial.

11:00 to 12:00 noon *Jojoba Hair and Scalp Conditioning Facial.* Put youthful brilliance and shine back into your hair with the natural oils of nature. This 30-minute conditioning treatment can transform your damaged hair into healthy looking hair.

Supplies

- Jojoba oil (if you cannot find jojoba oil you can use squalane)
- Macadamia nut oil
- Over-the-counter intensive hair conditioner
- Plastic shower cap or large towel
- Shampoo

Step One: Preparation. Mix 5 drops of jojoba or squalane oil and 4 drops of macadamia nut oil into 3 ounces of hair conditioner then mix well.

Step Two: Conditioning. Shampoo hair; then remove excess moisture with a towel. Apply the oil-enriched conditioner to your damp hair, then massage into hair and scalp to ensure complete coverage. Wrap hair in towel or cover with plastic shower cap and leave on for 40 minutes, then rinse well with warm water. Style your hair as usual.

12:00 to 1:00 P.M. *Gentle Facial, Throat, and Décolleté Skin Polishing.* Slough away unwanted dead skin cells with this skin polishing treatment. Your skin will feel as smooth as silk, and your complexion will glow.

Supplies

- Headband
- Cleanser
- Natural-bristle complexion brush
- Toner
- Facial Scrub
- Masque (the masque you use for your particular skin type)
- Moisturizer

Step One: Stimulating and deep cleansing. Pull back hair with the headband. Splash warm water onto your face, throat, and décolleté then apply cleanser to moistened areas. Moisten facial brush with water, then apply cleanser to the bristles. Begin at the base of your décolleté and work your way up to your forehead. Use a circular motion with a minimal amount of pressure. Remember, you're not scrubbing the floor. Also, avoid your eye area. Rinse with warm water.

Step Two: Exfoliating. While skin is still moist apply your facial scrub to your face, throat, and décolleté and gently massage with small circular motions. Begin at the base of the décolleté and work your way up, finishing at your forehead. Avoid eye area and do not tug or pull at your skin. Rinse well with warm water. (Please note if you have acne skin eliminate this step. If you have sensitive skin mix your facial scrub with 2 parts cleanser, it will be gentler on your complexion.)

Step Three: Skin softening. Massage a few drops of pure squalane or any light unscented face oil over entire area. Then apply your facial masque over the oil. Keep masque on for 20 minutes and relax in a reclining position with your feet elevated. After 20 minutes rinse well with warm water. Then splash face with toner if available and apply your day moisturizer while skin is still moist.

1:00 to 2:00 P.M. *Spa Lunch.* Lunch is on! Compliments of Kathy Swift, nutritionist for the Canyon Ranch Spa, Lenox, Massachusetts. Indulge yourself with a Delicious Vegetarian Pizza (255 calories), mixed green salad with nonfat bottled salad dressing (40 calories) and fresh sliced strawberries (1 cup 60 calories) for dessert. Both of these recipes are rich in nutrients that are good for the skin; the salad is packed with iron and calcium and the pizza is rich in antioxidants. See Chapter Four for recipes.

2:00 to 3:00 P.M. *Rosewater Spa Manicure.* Perfect pampering for your 10 little fingers. Discover how to give special attention to your hands and cuticles. Bathing your hands in delicious rosewater will help revive even the most abused hands.

Supplies

- Small kitchen bowl
- Nonacetone polish remover
- Medium-grade file
- Fine-grade file
- Smooth-grade file
- Pumice stick and pumice stone
- Rose oil
- Almond oil
- Facial scrub
- Natural-bristle nail brush
- Base polish, nail polish, and top coat

Step One: Preparation. Fill bowl with warm water and add 3 drops of rose oil.

Step Two: Correcting nail shape and surface. With the nonacetone nail-polish remover wipe away all the old nail polish. Use your medium-grade file to shape your nails. Take the fine-grade file and smooth the edges of your nails. If you have ridges on your nails take the nail buffer and use a short, gentle stroke to buff the tops of your nails. Buff your nails only in one direction and do not exceed 10 strokes per nail.

Step Three: Soak and exfoliate. Soak your hands and nails in the warm rosewater for 5 minutes. Then gently scrub under your nails with the natural-bristle nail brush. While your skin is still moist gently push back your cuticles with the pumice stick and then with the cuticle nipper gingerly cut off any hangnails or rough edges on your cuticles. Then take the pumice stone, moisten it with the water in the bowl, and gently buff any calluses or rough spots you may have on your hands. Take a nickel-size portion of facial scrub and massage both hands for about a minute or two, then rinse well.

Step Four: Conditioning. Massage both hands with sweet almond oil. Apply a little extra oil to all the nails and cuticles. Slip both hands into white cotton gloves and leave on for 30 minutes. While you are wearing the gloves, relax and listen to soothing music.

Step Five: Cosmetic care for the nails. Remove gloves and wipe off oil from each nail with a piece of cotton that is slightly moistened with nonacetone nail-polish remover. Apply a base coat to all your nails. Then apply nail polish to each nail. Try using the three-stroke method of applying nail polish: one down the center, then one on each side of the nail. Let dry, then apply a second coat of polish if you like. Add a top coat. Clean up the nail polish around your fingers by dipping an orangewood stick in nonacetone nail-polish remover and carefully cleaning around the cuticles.

3:00 to 5:00 P.M. *Escape for two hours.* Now is the time to do something nice for yourself. Why not have a professional massage? It's perfect for total relaxation. Schedule the appointment in advance for your spa weekend. You can even have the certified massage therapist come to your home for either a 1/2-hour or 1-hour massage. It's worth it.

5:00 to 7:00 P.M. *Spa Dinner.* Broiled Grouper with Tarragon Lime Sauce (only 225 calories) served with Boiled Red Bliss Potatoes (2 small 80 calories) and steam broccoli (1/2 cup 35 calories) is on the menu this evening, compliments of Kathy Swift, nutritionist for the Canyon Ranch Spa, Lenox, Massachusetts. This protein- and mineral-rich dinner offers you a well-balanced meal without a lot of calories. And, as a special treat for dessert try the Oatmeal Crumb Cake (130 calories). See Chapter Four for recipes.

7:00 to 9:00 P.M. *Dead Sea Mud Body Wrap and Warm Herbal Soak and Cool Shower.* This is a true spa treatment at its best. The unique mud used for this treatment is from Israel's Dead Sea, which offers many mineral-rich benefits to the skin. Enjoy the mud wrap, herbal soak, and invigorating cool shower. Your skin will feel as smooth as silk and your mood will be serene after this treatment.

Supplies

- Dead Sea mud (you can locate this product in many departments and health-food stores)
- 3 drops juniper oil, 6 drops peppermint oil, and 4 drops lavender oil
- Thin plastic sheet (this is used to wrap your body while the mud is on your body)
- Old sheet
- Warm thermal blanket
- Natural-bristle brush with 10″ handle
- Unscented body lotion

Step One: Preparation. *Your bed:* As a precaution so you do not soil your good bedding with the mud, you should remove the bedspread or comforter from your bed. First lay the old sheet on your bed, then the thermal blanket and then the plastic sheet.

Your bath: Fill your tub with warm water and add 3 drops of juniper oil, 6 drops of peppermint oil, and 3 drops of lavender oil.

Your body: Pull your hair up or wrap it in a towel. Take your natural-bristle body brush and gently stroke your skin with the brush by applying moderate pressure while your skin is dry. Begin this brushing technique at your feet and work your way up your thighs, buttocks, torso, and then your arms.

Step Two: Relaxing. Soak and relax for 20 minutes in the tub in the water that has been enriched with the essential oils.

Step Three: Conditioning. While still in the tub drain the water. Then while standing apply the mud all over your body while your skin is still moist. Begin at your ankles and work upward. Now run to your bed and lie on top of the plastic sheet. Then wrap yourself in the plastic sheet, thermal blanket, and old sheet that are laid out on the bed. Close your eyes and relax for 30 minutes.

Step Four: Conditioning. Unwrap yourself from the sheets and take a cool shower to rinse all the mud off your body. You might need the natural-bristle brush to help remove the mud. Pat skin dry with a large terry towel. Then massage your favorite lotion all over your body. Slip into something comfortable for bed.

9:00 to 10:00 P.M. *Quiet Time.* We all need time out, especially at the end of the day. Quiet time before you go to bed can become a valuable sleeping tool. It allows you to unwind from the day. Utilize this time in a positive way: read a book, listen to music, catch up on your letter writing. Quiet time is like a time out, so be good to yourself.

SUM IT UP!

The purpose of turning your home into a spa for a weekend is more than just beauty treatments—it is an exercise that can teach you how to be good to yourself. All the exotic treatments, advice, and delicious spa recipes are designed to help you discover the many new avenues that can renew your energy, help you eat nutritionally, and care for your skin from the tip of your head to your toes. Do the at-home spa weekend alone or with a spouse or friend—either way, you will laugh, you will relax, you will become spoiled. But most important, you will have done something special for yourself. You deserve it!

CHAPTER *Six*

CREATE AN AROMATHERAPY OASIS AT HOME

Imagine how amazed Cleopatra would be to discover that her beauty rituals of aromatherapy have become popular treatments in today's spas and salons. Aromatherapy has been embraced by many as a holistic beauty/health therapy in recent years, but this type of treatment is anything but new. In fact, it is one of the oldest forms of medicinal and beauty remedies and dates as far back as 3,000 to 5,000 B.C.

What does this curious word actually mean? Let's dissect it: "Aroma" means "agreeable odor" and "therapy" means "a treatment" or "intended to remedy or alleviate a disorder or an undesirable condition." Thus, aromatherapy is a healing treatment that utilizes aromatic essences, specifically, those found in plants. It is considered both an art and a science that taps directly into two important senses: touch and smell. This explains why using aromatic essences is not only good for the skin, but it also can help alter your mood in a positive way. The tension of a stressful day at the office, exam time at school, traffic jams, and long lines at the supermarket can be reduced through the use of pleasant aromas and massage.

Aromatherapy is personally delightful, but essential oils also have many medicinal properties and applications. The study of holistic, medical, and aesthetic aromatherapy is so immense it can take an aromatherapist (person who professionally practices aromatherapy) years to learn this science. Even after aromatherapists complete their schooling, an apprenticeship program may be necessary to gain all the knowledge it takes to safely practice the holistic and medical aspect of this science.

This chapter will address only the external application of aromatherapy as it pertains to maintaining beauty and reducing stress, not the internal or medical aspect of this subject. You will learn how the science of aromatherapy began, how essential oils are extracted from the plants, and about the power of these pure plant essences. You will discover how essential oils relate to the skin. You will also learn how to use these natural essences as a face splash, in a massage, in the shower or bath, and how to create your own "aromatherapy retreat." All of these holistic treatments will help you unwind from the vigorous demands of your daily activities.

GUESS WHAT! YOU'VE BEEN USING ESSENTIAL OILS AND YOU DIDN'T EVEN KNOW IT

To some people the whole concept of aromatherapy and the use of essential oils may sound mystical and full of "old wives tales." But for years, a few essential oils have been finding their way into mainstream products for their antiseptic, deodorizing, calming, or mentholated properties. For a point of reference I have listed some examples of products that use essential oils. Review the following list to see if you have ever used essential oils in some form or another. You may be surprised.

- Peppermint has been used in toothpastes, mouthwashes, and soaps for its clean, fresh scent and its incredible antiseptic properties that kill bacteria.
- Eucalyptus and its antiseptic and mentholated action has found its way into cough drops and inhalation remedies for colds and flus because of its decongestant action. It is a strong anti-bacteria agent so it helps stop the spread of germs. In the past surgeons have even used eucalyptus as a post-surgical dressing for incisions.

- Rose and its moisturizing properties have been used in one of the earliest skin preparations — rosewater and glycerin.
- Pine with its clean, fresh forest aroma and lemon with its zesty scent are two powerful deodorizers and antiseptics. These two oils were used in their natural form years ago in household cleaners. In recent years many companies have switched to a synthetic pine and lemon scent. But there are still a few environmentally conscious companies that use the "all natural" version of the pine and lemon essential oils.
- Essential oils with floral, spicy, woodsy, citrus, herbaceous scents are found in the more expensive perfumes.
- Many skin-care products such as cleansers, toners, moisturizers, and night cremes are tapping into the benefits of essential oils by incorporating them into their formulations.
- The more expensive candles, potpourri, sachets, and scented drawer liners all use essential oils to fill your house with their incredible aromas.
- Cedarwood chests, cedar-lined closets, and cedar balls and blocks (used for drawers and storage) have been used for hundreds of years for their cedarwood essential oil that repels insects such as moths and carpenter ants.
- Citronella (an essential oil with a slightly sweet, lemony aroma) candles have been used for many years to repel mosquitoes.

Are you surprised how many products contain aromatic essences oils? Now maybe essential oils won't seem so foreign to you as we discuss the therapeutic value of aromatherapy in this chapter.

FUN HISTORICAL FACTS ABOUT ESSENTIAL OILS

Ancient societies did not have the luxury of prepared medicines and toiletries as we do today. Our ancestors had to call upon the power of nature and what it produced: trees, plants, flowers, roots, seeds, and nuts. Through trial and error over the coarse of thousands of years they discovered the healing and beautifying virtues of plants. Experience taught them that some plants aided digestion; some were poisonous, and others offered healing properties (example; aloe vera soothes a burn). They steadily learned how the body was influenced by certain plants and flowers. To treat a burn, for example, they learned to pick a few leaves from an aloe vera plant or flower petals of lavender, rub them together to crush the leaves or petals and release the internal fluid of the plant. This fluid was then applied directly to the burn. They also burned aromatic plants; some smoke promoted a drowsy or calm feeling and other smoke produced an invigorating sensation.

The Egyptians continued and improved the use of aromatic plants. They learned how to extract a concentration of natural essences from the plant (the essential oils) by placing the plant material in oil or wine. It was during the fourth century B.C. that the Egyptians became familiar with the art and science of essential oil extraction. This ancient Egyptian aromatic custom was held in high esteem and kept a closely guarded secret. This new science was first dispensed only by high priests in religious ceremonies and embalming rituals. Bark such as cedarwood, resins such as frankincense, seeds such as caraway, and roots such as ginger were put into wine or oil. The aromatics would slowly steep and diffuse out and mix with the liquids. As the use of aromatics became more popular, they were prescribed by physicians as a medicine. And later only the very upper class could partake of these therapeutic plant essences.

The Hebrew, Greek, Arabic, Chinese, and Indian civilizations also utilized aromatic substances (essential oils) as an important part of their culture. These ancient civilizations used perfumed oils, scented spices, resins, and barks as well as aromatic vinegars, wines and beers. Their aromatics were used in embalming, religious rituals, medicine, beauty treatments, and astrology. In these cultures, males were as luxuriously perfumed as females.

AROMATIC ESSENCES—THE PERFECT STRESS-REDUCING REMEDY

Primitive peoples relied heavily on their sense of smell; it was key to survival. They used it to track animals and to determine if danger was close. Our sense of smell has been somewhat suppressed because of air pollution (especially car fumes, industrial waste chemical cleaning products, and artificial-fragrance room deodorizers, but even with all these factors working against us, our sense of smell remains quite acute 24 hours a day.

The area of our brain that houses our sense of smell and aroma has an incredible memory. It conjures up not just the visual memory, but also evokes the emotion that was felt at the time. That's why a whiff of a loved one's perfume will trigger a comforting and soothing response.

Our sense of smell is 10,000 times more sensitive than our sense of taste. Each of the nerves in the nose has a direct connection to the brain. This is why our sense of smell can compute and transmit the information with great speed. The sense of touch, sound, and taste communicates to the brain in a much more indirect fashion.

Aromatherapy utilizes our marvelous sense of smell. It uses scents such as lavender to soothe us when we're mentally fatigued and scents such as peppermint to perk us up and revive us. At the same time its oils pamper and nourish our skin. It's time to integrate the power of these abundant oils into your daily routine.

WHAT IS AN ESSENTIAL OIL?

Essential oils are the aromatic substances that are found in both cultivated and wild plants. They are called "volatile" liquids because they evaporate when exposed to the air. The survival of the plant depends on this substance: to attract pollinating insects, to influence growth and production, to protect itself from disease, to repel predators. This is where the name essential oil received its name because it is "essential" to the life of the plant. These natural essences accumulate in special cells of the plant that hold these precious essences. Essential oils may be found in the petals (lavender), the leaves (basil), the wood (cedarwood), the fruit (orange), the seeds (sesame), the roots (ginger), the gum (myrrh), the resin (pine), and in many cases it is located in more than one part of the plant. (An orange, for example, has essential oils in the white flowers, the rind, and the leaves.)

The chemistry of essential oils is complex. An essential oil consists of hundreds of components such as aldehydes, alcohols, terpene, and esters and there are also many undiscovered components. All of these aromatic substances are antiseptic in nature (eucalyptus and tea-tree have extraordinary antiseptic strength); some are endowed with anti-inflammatory properties (chamomile and lavender, for example) and anti-bacterial and anti-viral properties (as in garlic).

There are a number of factors that determine the efficacy of an essential oil: climate, altitude, soil conditions, and most important, when the plants are harvested. The level of this aromatic essence fluctuates during the day and night and with temperature. In most plants, warm weather induces a high concentration of this substance so this is the most favorable time for the gathering. But there are also a variety of night-scented flowers (jasmine, for example) that should be collected in the evening or at sunset.

An essential oil does not really have an oily texture. Actually, it is the complete opposite of an oil because it is not heavy or greasy. This substance, which is highly volatile (meaning it evaporates quickly), feels as light to the touch as water or alcohol. It disappears almost instantly when it is applied to the skin. If you were to place a drop of essential oil on a piece of paper it would not leave a permanent mark as a drop of regular oil would because regular oils are heavier in consistency and do not evaporate quickly.

Essential oils are an extremely concentrated substance, so a little goes a long way. But the cost varies depending on availability. There are some plants that have an abundance of this aromatic essence, making them inexpensive to purchase; then there are other varieties of plants that have only a scant amount of the essence, which makes them very expensive. For example, it takes 100 kilos of rose petals to yield a half liter of essential oil (very expensive type) while 100 kilos of lavender yields 3 liters of essential oil (more reasonably priced).

The fact that essential oils are so concentrated makes it necessary to mix and dilute them with what is called a carrier or base oil. Some excellent oils for this purpose (which also keep the skin soft and smooth) are: squalene oil, jojoba oil, rice bran oil, macadamia nut oil, almond oil, and apricot kernel oil. You do not apply an essential oil directly to the skin (unless directed by an experienced aromatherapist) because it could cause an irritation. You know the expression: *If a little is good, more doesn't mean it's better.* Well this holds true with essential oils because even though it is an excellent treatment you have to use it with care.

Six Methods to Extract Precious Essential Oils from Plants

The extraction process of an essential oil is extremely important because this affects the end product and determines its quality. There are several methods of extraction: ancient Egyptian clay-pot method, steam distillation, vacuum distillation, expression, enfleurage, and the volatile solvent extraction method, which is used in the perfume industry.

The ancient Egyptian clay-pot method is a classic technique of direct distillation. The material of the plant is placed directly in a water-filled still. When the water is heated the essential oils from the plant material are carried by the steam into the condenser (which cools the steam), and a separator separates the water from the essential oil.

Steam distillation is a much more effective procedure than the ancient, almost obsolete clay-pot method. Steam distillation eliminates the burning of the plant material in the distillation receptacle. In fact, the plant material is never in contact with the water; the steam just passes over it.

Vacuum distillation is a fairly new method. The sealed distillation apparatus has the air pressure reduced to create a vacuum. This allows distillation to occur at a much lower temperature. Preservation of the natural fragrance of the flower blossoms or plant material is accomplished much more effectively with this method than with steam distillation without the vacuum.

Expression is the least complicated of all the techniques of extraction. Pressure (exerted through centrifugal force) is applied to the plant to extract the aromatic substance.

Enfleurage is an almost obsolete method. A fatty oil (such as olive or sesame oil) is mixed with the plant material to absorb the essential oils and then separated from the fat by alcohol. Evaporation of the alcohol leaves only the essential oil behind.

Volatile solvent extraction is used often by the perfume industry. The two most popular solvents used for this purpose are liquid carbon dioxide and liquid butane. This method produces an exquisite true-to-life fragrance as it is found in nature.

Essential Oil Selection

There are hundreds of essential oils on the market today. To keep your initial exposure to aromatherapy simple, I've selected a limited variety of 20 essential oils for you to choose from, and all are readily available in specialty aromatherapy stores/salons, body and bath shops, and some department stores. This list of essential oils represents a good cross section of diverse actions (calming, energizing, refreshing, purifying, and cooling).

But which one is right for you? It depends actually on how you are going to use it. If you are going to use an essential oil on your face, the selection should be made according to skin type (oily, normal, dry), and if it is going to be used for relaxation purposes (as in a body massage, bath, or in an aromatherapy diffuser) then you should select the oils according to your state of mind and mood. If, for example, you felt you needed to be soothed because you were stuck in traffic and feeling a little nervous and uptight, chamomile essential oil would be a good choice because it has a soothing action.

The following information lists 20 essentials and a few base/carrier oils (these oils are used to dilute the essential oil). Discover where these essential oils originated from, the history behind the plant and the essential oil, and the action of these aromatic substances.

A QUICK GUIDE TO 20 POPULAR SKIN-RENEWING ESSENTIAL OILS FROM AROUND THE WORLD

Many essential oils have been used for thousands of years for their unique fragrances and healing properties. Learning about the origins and the ancient medicinal, ritualistic, and superstitious use of these aromatics is a fun way of becoming acquainted with these substances.

Bergamot: The name of the Bergamot tree comes from the small town of Bergamo in northern Italy. This is where the Bergamot tree (*Citrus Bergamia*) was originally cultivated. The part of the tree that is used for the essential oil is the rind of the fruit, which resembles a miniature orange. The aroma is an uplifting, clean citrus scent. Bergamot has powerful antiseptic and cooling properties so it is excellent for inflamed, irritated, and even blemished skin. It is important to keep in mind that Bergamot can cause photosensitivity so avoid the sun and tanning salons while using this oil.

Chamomile: This herb is cultivated in Morocco, Germany, and France, but it originated in Great Britain. There are two types of chamomile: Roman and German. Both contain an ingredient called Azulene that makes chamomile a powerful anti-inflammatory agent. This is a familiar herb because chamomile has been used as a tea to aid digestion and to calm nervousness and to induce a peaceful night's sleep. The essential oil in chamomile also has an analgesic action that helps to soothe inflamed or sensitive skin, burned or ruddy-looking skin, and blemished skin.

Cypress: This Mediterranean cone-shaped tree is part of the evergreen family. The part of the tree that is used for the essential oil are the cones, branches, and leaves. The aroma of cypress essential oil is woody and slightly spicy, yet refreshing. Cypress has a soothing and calming effect on your state of mind, and it has a balancing and equalizing effect on the skin.

Eucalyptus: Native to Austria, eucalyptus is a tree that is part of the evergreen family. In California, Florida, and in southern parts of the United States, the blue gum species of eucalyptus can be found. The eucalyptus bears a hard capsulelike fruit. The part of the tree that is used for essential oil is the mature leaves. Eucalyptus is familiar to most because it has been used in over-the-counter cough drops and as a decongestant for many years. It is also used worldwide as an inhalant for colds and the flu. It not only helps to open the nasal passages but it acts as an anti-bacterial and anti-viral agent helping to stop the spread of germs. There have been many surgeons who have used eucalyptus solution for its powerful antiseptic qualities in the operating room to flush out surgical wounds;

it has also been used as part of a post-operative dressing on surgical incisions. The scent is unforgettable because it has a penetrating, refreshingly crisp aroma. This essential oil's incredible antiseptic and bactericidal properties make this an excellent oil for blemished, burned, and inflamed skin. This oil also produces a cooling sensation on the skin.

Fennel: Native to the Mediterranean area and Asia, fennel is also cultivated in Europe and in the United States. The root of fennel has been used in many cultures as a vegetable, and the seeds have been used as a flavorful seasoning. The root and the seeds are also the parts used to obtain the essential oil. Fennel has a fresh, clean licorice aroma. Fennel tea has been used for thousands of years as a digestive remedy because it has a detoxifying effect. The cleansing and purging properties of this essential oil make it an excellent cleansing tool for all skin types.

Geranium: The two main sources for this essential oil are Morocco and an island in the southwestern Indian Ocean called Bourbon. In addition, essential oil is derived from the flower and leaves of a geranium called *Pelargonium Odorantissimum* (the one commonly found in window boxes). The scent of this essential oil is both sweet and heavy, like a rose, with an extremely light, refreshing overtone. Geranium essential oil is good for most skin because of the equalizing effect it has on sebum. Stimulating in action, it can help underactive, sluggish, and clogged skin.

Jasmine: This flower is native to the warmer parts of Iran and India, but it is also cultivated in Algeria, Morocco, Egypt, Italy, and the southern United States. Jasmine, like rose, is a very costly essential oil because large quantities of the branches and petals need to be distilled to produce a small quantity of the exquisite essential oil. The aroma of this essence is exotic and sweet. Jasmine has been called the "king of flowers" because in ancient times it was used as an aphrodisiac. Many ceremonial rituals in India used jasmine. In China the stems were used to make jasmine tea, and it is used as a food garnish in Indonesia. Jasmine's rich moisturizing properties make it an excellent oil for dry, mature, and sun-damaged skin.

Juniper: This native Scandinavian evergreen shrub thrives in articlike conditions, but it is also found in many parts of the world. With needlelike leaves and blue-black berries, juniper has a slightly woody yet refreshing aroma. In the late eighteen hundreds, French hospitals used to burn juniper and rosemary to cleanse the air of germs. The purifying effect of this essence helps most skin types but especially oily, blemished skin with clogged pores.

Lavender: This is probably one of the most popular oils ever used. The Romans used lavender to wash with and also tend to any sores; the French aristocrats used lavender as a mouthwash. For ages it has been used as a sachet in closets and drawers because it helps to repel moths and other insects. The analgesic properties of lavender kill bacteria on the skin as they help to soothe and reduce inflammation. The scent of this essential oil is a clean, light floral aroma with a woody overtone that is extremely comforting and soothing to one's state of mind.

Lemon: This irregularly shaped tiny evergreen tree was originally native to India but is now abundant in California, Florida, and in southern Europe. The essential oil is obtained from the fruit and peel of the lemon. The citrus aroma is clean and fresh, yet sharp. The pore-cleansing action of this essence makes it therapeutic for all skin types but especially those that are oily.

Marjoram: Sweet marjoram originates in Egypt and the Mediterranean. The ancient Greeks valued the medicinal qualities of this herb, which they used to calm muscle spasms, reduce excess fluid, and camouflage odor. Marjoram has also been used as a subtle seasoning for foods. With a slightly spicy, warm, penetrating aroma it has a calming effect on your state of mind. The analgesic action of marjoram can benefit a sensitive and inflamed skin.

Neroli: The essential oil derived from the white flowers of an orange tree found in China received its name after the Countess of "Neroli" used the aromatic essences to perfume her bath water and her clothing. The tree can also be found in Morocco, Italy, Portugal, and France. The intriguing floral fragrance is derived from the white petals of the flowers. The scent is somewhat hypnotic, which helps to relieve stress and anxiety. Dry and mature skin benefit a great deal from this moisturizing oil.

Orange: The orange tree was native to China and India, but it was then cultivated in Europe during the seventeenth century. As you know, it is grown in the United States and is also found in the Mediterranean region and Israel. Three different essential oils are obtained from three parts of the tree: orange essential oil is obtained from the rind; neroli from the white flowers; petitgrain from the leaves. Orange essential oil has a refreshing yet zesty aroma.

Patchouli: This bush plant with purple-hue and white flowers is native to India, Paraguay, Burma, and Malaysia and is the main source for the essential oil that is obtained from the young leaves. It was common practice in ancient India to perfume drawer liners with patchouli sachets. The scent was used to keep moths away from the cashmere shawls made in India during the turn of the century. It has a powerful, exotic, earthy aroma that is also spicy and sweet and that gets deeper and fuller as it ages. Patchouli cools an inflamed skin condition, and it helps to heal and soften rough, cracked skin.

Pine: Found in Scandinavia, East Russia, and Northern Europe, this tree has approximately 75 to 85 species. The two varieties that are usually used for obtaining essential oil from the bark, needles, and the cone are the Norwegian and the Scots Pine. In ancient times it was used as an inhalation therapy for respiratory ailments. Native American tribes of North America drank an infusion (tealike drink) of the vitamin-C-rich pine needle because it helped to ward off scurvy (a vitamin C deficiency). Today this essential oil is used in a variety of products such as soaps and bath salts because of its deodorizing properties. The clean, fresh forest fragrance helps to revive mental fatigue. The antiseptic qualities help to cleanse the skin and kill bacteria.

Rose: The most popular sources for rose essential oil are France, Turkey, Morocco, and Bulgaria. This is an extremely expensive oil because it takes many flowers to make a small amount of the essential oil. The sweet floral aroma has made this essence popular in the perfume industry. The scent of the rose is extremely soothing and helps to relieve stress. One of the first skin preparations used to soften the skin was made out of roses and called rosewater and glycerin. The moisturizing properties of rose oil helps to soften dry, mature, sun-damaged, and sensitive skin. It leaves the skin feeling silky smooth.

Rosemary: This herb originated in Asia, but it is grows abundantly in the Mediterranean, France, and Yugoslavia. This was considered a sacred plant to the ancient Greeks, Romans, and Egyptians because a superstitious belief said it gave peace to the living and the deceased. It was also used as a facial wash by Donna Isabella, Queen of Hungary. French hospitals in the eighteenth century used rosemary incense for its antiseptic properties. Rosemary also has been used by many to season meats, vegetables, and breads. The crisp, penetrating, powerfully refreshing herbal aroma has a stimulating action that helps to increase alertness and revive mental fatigue. The deep cleansing and antiseptic action of rosemary helps to kill bacteria on the skin and helps to soften the debris that is found in clogged pores. The stimulating action of this herb is invigorating to the skin, especially to underactive, dull complexions.

Sandalwood: This evergreen tree native to India doesn't mature until it reaches 60 years of age. The fragrant essence is obtained from the inner wood of the tree. In ancient times sandalwood was used to build furniture because it would resist and repel insects. Sandalwood incense was used during prayer and meditation in ancient India, Greece, Egypt, and Rome because it had a calming effect. The ancient Egyptians used it for embalming purposes because it helped prevent decomposition. The lingering woody, sweet, somewhat exotic fragrance helps to soothe nerves and gives a peaceful feeling. The rejuvenating and preserving action of this essence helps to smooth and soften dry, mature, sun-damaged skin. Its antiseptic qualities help kill bacteria on the skin, and its soothing action helps relieve inflammation and reduce ruddiness.

Tea-Tree: Similar to the cypress tree, this evergreen, native to South Wales, flourishes in marshy areas. The essential oil is produced in Australia from both the wood and the leaves. Wounds of the Australian Aborigines were treated with tea-tree essential oils.

The antiseptic qualities also made this a popular medicinal remedy during World War II. The first-aid medical kits contained essence of tea-tree, which was to be used as a topical antiseptic. It has been used frequently in deodorants and soaps, as well as surgical and dental supplies. The pungent, fresh, clean-smelling aroma refreshes and revitalizes your state of mind. As an antiseptic it kills bacteria on the skin and quickly reduces inflammations, and its warm, sometimes tingling sensation can soothe tired, aching muscles.

Ylang Ylang: This small tropical tree is found in the South Sea islands and has pink, mauve, and yellow flowers. It was called "The Perfume Tree" because the women of these islands used to perfume their hair with the aromatic essences from the tree. In ancient times, Indonesians placed petals on the sheets of the bed on their wedding night to fragrance them. The exotic, rich, sweet floral aroma has been described as seductive and relaxing. Both oily skin and dry skin can benefit from this oil because it has an equalizing effect on the complexion.

IMPORTANT TIPS TO PRESERVE THE STRENGTH OF YOUR ESSENTIAL OILS

Essential oil is packaged in glass because pure essential oils can break down many types of plastic material. The glass is usually amber colored because the dark glass protects the volatile essential oil from sunlight, which can affect its composition. If you transfer your essential oils into another container make sure it is a dark-colored glass. And always keep your essential oils in a cool, dark place. You want to avoid direct contact with the sun in order to preserve the quality and effectiveness of the essence.

ESSENTIAL OILS AND NATURAL SKIN-SOOTHING OILS—A PERFECT TEAM

Essential oils are too concentrated to use directly on the skin. When using these essences in massage it's necessary to use a substance to dilute their power. The perfect substance to dilute an essential oil is an unscented lubricating oil such as sweet almond oil, squalene, sunflower oil, safflower oil, soy oil, jojoba oil, macadamia nut oil, apricot kernel oil, or grapeseed oil. These oils are called carrier or base oils because they are the vehicle that holds the active ingredient (the essential oil) in the recipe or formulation. Besides diluting the essential oils these therapeutic plant oils help provide a slippery surface so the movement of the massage stroke can slide almost frictionlessly across the skin. An added benefit of these oils comes from the essential fatty acids they contain, which help soften the skin and provide a thin barrier to hold in moisture.

If you'd rather not mix your own essential oils, you can buy preblended ones that are already labeled for appropriate use such as "relaxing," "invigorating," and so on.

Safety Guidelines for Using Essential Oils at Home

- Never use an essential oil directly on the skin. It is important to dilute it either in one of the carrier/base oils or in water. (Note: Water is not a good vehicle for a massage.)
- If you are pregnant, you should avoid these essential oils because they are strong oils and have not been tested on skin affected by the hormonal changes of pregnancy: basil, clove, hyssop, marjoram, and myrrh.
- These oils are not safe for home use because they are exceptionally strong: wintergreen, thyme, sage, and origanium.
- These oils should not be used on the skin because they may cause irritation: cinnamon, clove.
- These oils cause photosensitivity (a sensitive reaction to the sun that causes the skin to burn and become irritated) and should not be applied to the skin before you expose yourself to the sun or tanning booth (both of which are hazardous to your skin): bergamot, orange, grapefruit, lemon, all citrus fruits, and verbena.

WATER THERAPIES—THE ART OF BATHING

Water therapy is a time-honored prescription. The ancient Egyptians and Romans made bathing an important part of their culture. In these societies a bath was not just a bath but a delightful and pleasurable series of bathing phases: First they immersed themselves in an invigorating hot bath for a short while (in many cases they may have used the hot water from a mineral spring); the second bath was tepid and for long, leisurely soaks; and the third and last bath was cold and enriched with the aromatic essences of essential oils. After this luxurious soak, they had a massage with aromatic essences.

Today, spas around the world take advantage of the therapeutic effects of water. Many spas use water therapies such as relaxing hydrotherapy as a prelude to the other treatments. (Hydrotherapy uses a special tub that has many water jets that cause a pulsating action against the skin.)

If your days are filled with stress, a "water therapy" bath can help you relax (even if it's only for 15 to 20 minutes a day). Soaking in warm water infused with aromatic essential oils may be just the prescription you need when you feel frazzled or drained of every ounce of energy.

Envision yourself slipping into a warm, fragrant bath. Now you take a deep breath so you can take in the inviting aroma. The water should be about the same as your body temperature (98.6 degrees) so you feel as if you're one with the water. You close your eyes while you soak in this precious aromatic fluid so you can completely detach from the events of the day. Sound too good to be true? It's not. This is probably one of the most convenient and inexpensive forms of relaxation therapy known today.

Water Therapy Recipes

The recipes for heightening the therapeutic value of your water experience are extremely simple to prepare. Each recipe takes only a few drops of undiluted oils added to your bath water.

The Refresher. 4 drops lemon, 2 drops geranium essential oil, juice from a half a grapefruit.

A.M. Energizer. 4 drops juniper, 3 drops peppermint, 4 drops lavender.

Nighttime Soother. 3 drops chamomile, 4 drops rose, 2 drops neroli.

Summer Cooler. 3 drops peppermint, 5 drops cypress, 3 drops lemon.

Mentholated Uplift. 3 drops eucalyptus, 3 drops pine, 2 drops lavender.

Suggestions to Maximize the Effectiveness of Your Bath

1. Never use extremely hot water. Rather than offer therapeutic benefits, a steaming bath drains every ounce of energy from your body. Lukewarm water is the best temperature for therapeutic value; because the water is close to your body's temperature it produces a relaxing and soothing action.
2. Add the essential oil to the bath while the water is running. Before you get into the tub swish the water around so the essential oils mix well with the water. Don't let too much time elapse between the time you add the oils and the time you enter the tub because the oils evaporate quickly and you don't want to lose their benefits.
3. If your skin is on the dry side, mix the essential oils with 1 ounce of a base/carrier oil such as pure squalene, sweet almond oil, jojoba, wheat-germ oil, or macadamia nut oil. Then add this mixture to the bath. And don't forget to swish the water before entering the tub so the oils mix with the water.
4. The purpose of the bath is to make you feel as if you are a thousand miles away in some secluded, special oasis. This atmosphere cannot be achieved if negative noise (traffic, sirens, loud conversations, and so on) slips into your space. Soft background music will help to drown out any undesirable sounds.
5. Close your eyes while you bathe. This is a very important part of your bath experience. When your eyes are closed you can shut out the world and really relax.
6. It's very important to care for your skin after your bath if you want your skin to hold onto the newly gained moisture and essential oils. Never get out of the bath and grab a towel and rub yourself dry because this defeats the purpose of the "water therapy" bath. While your skin is still wet from the bath apply

a rich body lotion, body milk, or body oil (you could add a drop or two of your favorite essential oil to a portion of your body product) and massage it into your moist skin. Then slip into an oversized, thick terry-cloth robe. The robe will absorb the excess moisture.

MASSAGE WITH ESSENTIAL OILS—THE PERFECT ANTIDOTE FOR STRESS

It is difficult to measure all the many benefits of touch. Besides being simply enjoyable and pleasurable, massage is a great way to release stress. When you combine massage with the use of aromatic essential oils you add another beneficial dimension: the sense of smell.

On a physical level massage offers many benefits. It provides stress reduction and deep relaxation, relief from muscle tension and stiffness, better circulation, tension relief, and nourished skin. Massage also delivers on a mental level. Massage will promote a calm state of mind, increase alertness, and reduce mental stress. Massage affects one's emotional level also. It produces a sense of well-being and reduced levels of anxiety.

Obviously, for many reasons, massage is a perfect way to begin or end your week.

Massage/Body Oil Recipes

What you place on the skin is an important aspect of massage, especially when you're introducing aromatherapy to the treatment. Natural body oils can relieve a whole host of skin symptoms: from dry, itchy, flaky skin to chapped and wind-burned skin to itchiness from soap irritation. The extremely light oil film from the product produces a thin barrier that protects your skin against loss of moisture. Here are a few luxurious, all-natural massage recipes that are easy to mix. You can use them as moisturizing body oils alone or with your massage.

How to mix the carrier/base oil In a small plastic bowl mix together the following: 1 ounce of avocado oil, 1 ounce of squalene oil, 1 ounce sweet almond oil. You can use this base oil with any of the following recipes. Please note: If it is difficult to find any of the above carrier/base oils, you can substitute them with any of the other lubricating oils. But keep in mind that wheat-germ oil (which happens to be a great oil because it's rich in antioxidant vitamin E) tends to be a bit sticky.

"Sore Muscle" Massage/Body Oil. Add the following essential oils directly to the prepared base oil: 7 drops chamomile, 4 drops lavender, 3 drops rosemary essential oil. Mix thoroughly.

"Citrus" Massage/Body Oil. Add the following essential oils directly to the prepared base oil: 6 drops lemon, 6 drops orange and 4 drops grapefruit essential oil. Mix thoroughly.

"Floral" Massage/Body Oil. Add the following essential oil directly to the prepared base oil: 4 drops jasmine, 2 drops rose essential oil. Mix thoroughly.

"Soothing" Massage/Body Oil. Add the following essential oil to the prepared base oil: 7 drops lavender, 3 drops chamomile, 4 drops marjoram essential oil. Mix thoroughly.

Massage Advice

1. The skin should be free of all products: oils, cremes, and lotions.
2. The atmosphere should be serene: dim the lights; turn off the phone; turn off the TV. Soft instrumental music should be playing in the background to drown out any undesirable noise.
3. Choose the appropriate massage oil recipe that best fits the mood at the moment (Are you stressed out? Overheated? Drained of energy?).
4. The oil should be slightly warmed. Before applying the oil, warm it in your hands.
5. The flow of the massage stroke should not be broken. Always keep one hand on the person at all times even if you need to add more massage oil. This helps to avoid the sudden stop and go action that could defeat the relaxing aspect of the massage.
6. Never pour the massage oil directly onto the person. Pour it into your hands first, and hold it there for a moment so the oil

absorbs the warmth from your hands. Then apply the oil to the person. Don't drown the skin with oil; apply only what you need for the area you are working on. You can always add more when you need to.

7. If you are inexperienced when it comes to performing a massage, it is best to keep your technique light to the touch. If the person that you are massaging shows signs of discomfort when you are massaging an area, it's best to ease the amount of pressure you are applying.
8. If the person has a sore spot, you can perform a localized massage on the problem area. But you should begin with the back, feet, or hands so that the person is relaxed before you reach the problem area.
9. Avoid showering up to three to four hours after an essential oil massage because you don't want to rinse away the therapeutic value of the oils. Slip into a terry-cloth robe and relax.

DAILY SKIN CARE WITH ESSENTIAL OILS

Aromatic Facial Waters

If you want to incorporate the use of essential oils into your daily skin-care routine, aromatic facial waters are the simplest way to begin. Water is an important component of any skin-care routine because it is used during your morning and evening skin-care program when you splash your face with water over and over. This special fluid helps to rehydrate your skin. Essential oils and water can team up to make an incredible skin treatment.

Aromatic Facial Water Recipes: Aromatic water is simple and inexpensive. First, select the essential oil recipe that best suits your skin. Then add it to running water as you fill your bathroom sink with approximately two cups of warm water.

Aromatic Water for Mature/Sun-damaged Skin. Add this essential oil recipe to the warm water: 2 drops geranium, 2 drops chamomile, 2 drops juniper essential. Swish the water around to thoroughly mix solution. Splash your face 10 to 15 times.

Aromatic Water for Inflamed Skin. Add this essential oil recipe to the warm water: 3 drops chamomile, 2 drops lavender essential oil. Swish the water around to thoroughly mix solution. Splash your face 10 to 15 times.

Aromatic Water for Oily Skin. Add this essential oil recipe to the warm water: 3 drops ylang ylang, 3 drops bergamot, 4 drops lavender essential oil. Swish water around to thoroughly mix solution. Splash your face 10 to 15 times.

Aromatic Water for Dry Skin. Add this essential oil recipe to the warm water: 3 drops sandalwood, 2 drops rose essential oil. Swish water around to thoroughly mix solution. Splash your face 10 to 15 times.

Aromatic Water for All Skin Types. Add this essential oil recipe to warm water: 5 drops lavender essential oil. Swish water around to thoroughly mix solution. Splash your face 10 to 15 times.

The aromatic water treatment can be done once or twice a day and can be used in place of a toner. After you finish splashing your face and while your skin is still moist apply your moisturizer or night creme.

Special little beauty tip: You could place one of the mixtures into a small atomizer so you can spritz your face during the day at home, in the office, or when you're traveling. The solution is good for only a couple of days.

Aromatic Facial Steam

You can deep-cleanse your skin with warm, moist, essential-oil-enriched steam. The therapeutic values of steam are many: It helps soften and rehydrate the outer layer (stratum corneum) of your skin; it helps unclog pores; the warmth of the steam stimulates circulation, making the skin look pink and rosy. When you add an essential oil mixture to the steam, you are boosting the benefits of the steam by addressing the needs of your skin type (oily, normal, dry, mature, sun-damaged).

(Even though steam has all these wonderful benefits it is not good for every skin type. If you have ruddy [red-looking], sensitive skin or severely inflamed acne you should not use this treatment.)

Supplies for Aromatic Facial Steam:
large kitchen bowl
large bath towel
essential oils of your choice

Directions:

Step One: Add a total of 12 drops of essential oil to 3 cups of water that was just boiled. (Add 4 drops at a time at 5-minute intervals.)

Step Two: Put a towel over your head like a tent so the steam is concentrated on the facial area and doesn't escape. Steam your face for approximately 15 minutes.

Recipes:

Aromatic Facial Steam for Mature and Sun-Damaged Skin. Use 6 drops patchouli, 6 drops lemon essential oil.

Aromatic Facial Steam for Sensitive Skin. Use 6 drops chamomile, 5 drops lavender essential oil.

Aromatic Facial Steam for Oily Skin. Use 6 drops fennel, 5 drops rosemary, 3 drops lemon essential oil.

Aromatic Facial Steam for Dry Skin. Use 4 drops sandalwood, 6 drops rose essential oil.

Aromatic Facial Steam for All Skin Types. Use 6 drops lavender, 6 drops lemon essential oil.

Beauty advice: It's nice to do a mild facial scrub and masque after a facial steam. After the steam, your skin has been deep-cleansed and rehydrated, making it extremely receptive to your skin-care products. (Complete details of facial scrubs and masques are in Chapter Three.)

FRESHEN YOUR ENVIRONMENT WITH ESSENTIAL OILS

Aromatherapy can definitely help freshen and cleanse the air in your home or workplace. Essential oils are much better than room deodorizers that mask the odor or may even contain artificial fragrances. Essential oils are completely natural, and they offer the added benefit of being able to help you set the appropriate mood at a moment's notice.

An aromatic essential oil diffuser is the most efficient way to dispense essential oil into the air. It is an electrical apparatus that gently mists the essential oil into the air. It can easily be installed in your home or office and can be purchased in specialty aromatherapy shops/salons and in some bath and body stores. The diffuser will help you create a pleasant atmosphere for very little cost. Follow the manufacturer's directions regarding the quantity of essential oils you should place into this apparatus.

If you don't want to purchase a diffuser, you can place a couple of drops of essential oil on a light bulb. The warmth of the bulb will speed up the evaporation process and disperse the essential oil into the air. Place two to three drops on the bulb while it is still cold. (Never place it on the light while it is hot.) The light-bulb technique is not as efficient as the diffuser, but it's a good way to experiment before you spend any money on a piece of equipment.

Here are a few essential oil suggestions that will help you choose an essestial oil to fit your mood. Select only one, two, or three essential oils out of a particular category to use at one time and follow the manufacturer's directions for the amount you need for the diffuser.

Purifier. Use pine, juniper, eucalyptus, bergamot, lemon, geranium, lavender essential oils.

Anti-Depressant. Use cedarwood, chamomile, sandalwood, geranium, rose essential oils.

Calming. (Great for the evening.) Use marjoram, chamomile, lavender, patchouli essential oils.

Stimulating. (Great for the morning.) Use peppermint, rosemary, pine essential oils.

To Calm Nervousness and Anxiety. Use neroli, marjoram essential oils.

To Promote Mental Alertness. Use peppermint, rosemary, juniper, orange essential oils.

SUM IT UP!

With essential oils you can renew a kinship with natural plants' essences as our ancestors once did. Aromatherapy can add a new dimension to your life by reviving your sense of smell, which has been anesthetized by the bombardment of daily pollution. Your sense of smell, your mood, your state of mind, and your skin can be influenced in a positive way by this completely natural fluid.

The subject of aromatherapy in its entirety is complex, but in this chapter you've been given a basic introduction to the easiest and safest ways to use essential oils in your daily life. You now know how to use these oils in your bath, in massage, in aromatic water for a facial splash, in facial steams, and as an environmental essence. I encourage you to enjoy all of the aromatic recipes that can help you either reduce your stress level, soothe your frazzled nerves, or give you vitality. Aromatherapy is a way of getting closer to nature because you are tapping into the "essential" substances that are crucial to the survival of the plants. I like to think of essential oils as "nature" captured in a bottle.

Part TWO

Special Considerations

CHAPTER *Seven*

JUST FOR MEN

For thousands of years men have enjoyed being pampered and well groomed—these pleasures are not for women only. In ancient times it was extremely popular and "politically correct" for men to take part in aromatic bathing and massage treatments. Japanese men enjoyed hot mineral baths, vigorous body brushing, and massage. The Roman baths were very popular in their time. This is where men would plunge into various pools of water that were regulated at different temperatures ranging from cold to warm to hot. (The hot baths contained aromatic essential oils.) Egyptian men would relax in an essential oil bath, which was followed by an aromatic massage. And aristocratic French men gargled with floral lavender water, wore face powder, and perfumed their handkerchiefs.

Even the barber shops of the more recent past were a haven for men and their grooming needs, offering a shave, a facial massage, a hot-towel compress, a manicure, and a haircut. Although the corner barber shops don't attract the crowds they used to, there are still many men who enjoy a shave or massage at the golf or athletic club. These grooming rituals give them a new lease on life.

So why should you limit yourself to just the daily shave, nail trim, and occasional haircut. It is perfectly acceptable to primp and groom yourself. In fact, today's competitive work environment demands that you put your best foot forward. If you have had a particular skin problem that has been bothering you, such as irritated skin from shaving, dry, flaky skin, excess oiliness, or callused hands, it is probably quickly and easily remedied.

Caring for your skin, hands, and feet doesn't have to take hours of time or tons of products. In many cases a skin-care treatment can be worked into your shaving routine without any fuss.

Men and women have the same needs when it comes to caring for the skin: proper cleansing, exfoliating, moisturizing, and protection from the sun. Be sure to read this entire book to learn about how your skin functions, how to recognize the type of skin you have, how to decide what type of products you need, how to feed your skin from within, how to protect your skin from the sun's UV rays, how to have a more youthful-looking complexion, and lots more. This chapter focuses on a few specialized skin-care treatments, shaving, and hand treatments that are most appropriate for men.

DOES YOUR BABY FACE HAVE THE SHAVING BLUES?

Every morning your razor blade travels across the sensitive living terrain of your face; it climbs mountains, valleys, and flat lands. If your razor blade isn't up to par for this journey, I hate to think what you're doing to your skin. Are razor burns, razor bumps, ingrown hair, irritation, nicks, or cuts common shaving hazards you've experienced? If you suffer from the "baby-face shaving blues," here are a few simple shaving survival tips that could save your delicate skin from common shaving dangers.

The Blade

Plastic disposable and refill cartridges are much more advanced and therefore more effective than the safety doubled-edged razor. The pivoting action of the cartridge type of razor offers easy jockeying over your skin. The blades that are coated last the longest and are the sharpest. Another shaving option is the electric razor, which doesn't give the closest shave, but is less likely to cause razor burns, cuts, or nicks. With an electric razor, your skin isn't in close contact with the blade because it is protected by the special shield on the head of the razor.

Proper Razor Maintenance Can Save Your Skin

A blade is not expected to last forever. Dull blades and rushing your shave are the primary causes of razor burn and nicks. If you change the blade once or twice a week you're guaranteed a sharp blade that will glide over your skin. When your blade is sharp you don't need to apply as much pressure. Don't use a towel to dry your blades, just rinse the blade and let it air dry. Touching the edge of the blade with anything like a towel damages the shaving edge, which lessens the life and efficiency of the blade. Also, sharing your razor is a real "no-no" because you lose track of how many times the blade was used.

Too Close for Comfort

Your quest for the closest, smoothest shave could be causing your skin to look and feel irritated and raw. Razor burn occurs when your blade takes a little more off your face than just your whiskers and dead skin cells. Facial abrasions are caused by a dull blade, unprepared skin, rushing, and applying too much pressure. Cutting too close also increases your chance of getting ingrown hair, nicks, and cuts.

The solution: A protective layer (and I'm not talking about soap) between your delicate skin and the cold, hard steel of your blade can prevent many shaving problems. A thin film of moisturizer and lubrication will do the trick. Use plenty of warm water to moisten the skin and soften your beard stubble. Next apply a thin film of rich moisturizer, then apply a conditioning type of shaving preparation. Then let it set for 5 minutes so you can maximize the softening benefits to the skin and your beard. That's all there is to it: a splash or two of water, a slap of moisturizer, and a few smears of conditioning shaving gel or creme and you're ready for a close, painless shave.

Shaving Bumps Ingrown hair is a common cause of an irritation due to shaving called shaving bumps. In African Americans, razor bumps, also known as "pseudofolliculitis," are a serious, scarring skin problem. Curved hair follicles are the cause. Instead of growing outward, the curve of the hair causes it to reenter the skin and become ingrown, which results in an inflammation. Shaving then aggravates the condition.

Solution: Growing a beard is the best solution but that may not always be feasible. You may have to experiment with your shaving method. Don't shave too closely, don't shave against the grain, and above all, use a sharp razor. If you are an African American you might want to try a chemical depilatory product that dissolves hair at the surface, causing less irritation to the follicle. If the condition worsens you should consult a dermatologist as soon as possible before the razor bumps leave permanent scars.

Easy Does It

Rushing through your shave could be hazardous to the health of your face and neck, especially if you are half asleep in the morning. If you can't be trusted not to hurt yourself with this sharp object (and you know who you are), then try shaving before your go to bed in the evening (of course this works only if you have a light beard). If this won't do the trick for you, then get up earlier and slow down.

Shaving Can Strip Away Precious Moisture

Why would you want to slap an after-shave lotion (which is loaded with alcohol) directly on your skin after you shave? Do you like the burn? There is no benefit to this treatment because it contributes to dry skin and aggravates any irritation you may have. When you finish your shave you should splash your face with plenty of warm water; then, while your skin is still moist, drench it with a water-based moisturizer. This will replenish the skin's natural oils you have shaved away.

Ouch! First Aid Suggestions

If you've had a little accident with your razor and you've given yourself a nick or a cut it's important to treat it immediately. When the bleeding stops apply an antibiotic ointment (which can be purchased in any pharmacy) directly to the problem area.

If your skin is irritated and you have to shave over it, try applying an over-the-counter topical cortisone cream first. Apply the cortisone cream before you apply your conditioning shaving preparation. The anti-inflammatory nature of this medicated cream will calm your skin while you shave. After a few days if you haven't gotten any relief and your skin is still irritated consult with a dermatologist as soon as possible because you could have a condition called foliculitis, which is a bacterial infection in the hair follicle.

Sensitive Skin Advice

Shaving in the direction your beard grows can save you from a great deal of pain and skin sensitivities. An over-the-counter cortisone cream can be applied under your shaving preparation before you shave to help reduce the chance of new irritations or razor burn. If you don't want to use cortisone you could try applying either a moisturizer with chamomile or an aloe vera gel under your shaving preparation before you shave and then again immediately after you shave. Both of these plant essences have anti-inflammatory properties. Also, a cool compress saturated in chamomile tea will help to reduce the uncomfortable burning sensation.

TWO UNSPOKEN PROBLEMS AND HOW TO CORRECT THEM

There are two sensitive issues that are not serious to your health but may concern you because they affect your appearance. They are (1) rough callused skin and (2) discolored fingernails. These problems can be an occupational or a recreational condition. Common causes are gardening, construction, painting, car maintenance, or simply doing lots of work with your hands. Even though your hands may look hopeless they're not. Read on and you will find two simple and inexpensive remedies that will help you whip into shape your callused skin or discolored nails.

Rx for Rough Callused Skin

Do your hands sometimes look and feel rough? Do your hobbies or your work make your hands look discolored and stained? Do they look the same no matter how many times you wash them? Here's a remedy that will do the trick.

Supplies:
3/4 cup coarse sea salt
1 ounce of sweet almond oil
3 tablespoons baking powder
3 drops lemon essential oil
small kitchen bowl
small cup (you can use a coffee cup)

Mixing directions: Pour 3/4 cup sea salt and 3 tablespoons baking powder into a bowl and mix these two ingredients together. In a small cup add 1 ounce of sweet almond oil and 3 drops of lemon essential oil and mix. Now add the mixed oils to the bowl with the salt/baking powder and mix.

Rub this aromatic salt mixture on the problem areas: callused hands, feet, elbows and/or knees. Always apply to skin that has been moistened with water and use a circular motion when massaging the mixture on your skin. Rinse and apply a rich body lotion or hand creme.

The friction of the salt will polish the skin to help slough off some of the callus, the oil will soften the skin, and the baking powder and the lemon essential oil will help to deodorize and lighten the stained skin. It may have taken years to build up these calluses so it may take a few treatments to whip your callused skin back into shape.

Remedy for Discolored Nails

Discolored nails are unsightly because even though your nails have been scrubbed they may still look unkempt. Here are a few quick tips that will help you shape up your nails and transform them from dingy to sparkling.

Supplies:
nail brush
small kitchen bowl
hydrogen peroxide (can be found in any pharmacy)
2 tablespoons of baking powder in a small bowl

Directions:

Step One: File down your nails to remove part of the stain. Then soak your nails in a small bowl filled with hydrogen peroxide for 5 minutes.

Step Two: Dip the moistened bristles of the nail brush into the bowl with the baking powder. The moisture from the brush will help to form a paste. Then brush this pasty mixture under and on top of your nails for a couple of minutes. Don't rinse yet, let this baking powder mixture sit on and under your nails for 10 minutes, then rinse.

The abrasiveness of the baking powder will help to buff away some of the stain and help to whiten your nails.

Tips to Help Prevent Fingernail Staining

This can be simpler than you think. Before you paint, garden, work on your car, or do any rough work with your hands, you should first moisturize your hands with a rich hand creme. Then take a bar of soap and run your nails over the top so the soap will collect under your nails. Then put on your work gloves. The soap, hand creme, and the work gloves will protect your hands and nails from the staining agents. And if you can't work with gloves just use the hand creme and the soap under your nails. When you finish working, take your nail brush and plenty of water and scrub away the soap under your nails. You can also avoid staining by applying a clear matte nail polish (it looks invisible on your nails because there is no shine); this helps to form an invisible barrier between you and the staining agent.

QUICK SKIN AND GROOMING TIPS

Neck Irritation

Does your shirt collar cause the skin around your neck to burn and look irritated? This is a common complaint among men, especially during the summer when there is increased perspiration. The front of your neck is shaved every day so the throat region may be sensitive to begin with; then when you combine the moisture from sweating (which is on the acidic side) with the friction of the skirt rubbing against the skin, you get a burning mess that is quite uncomfortable.

The Solution: Try dusting your throat area and the inside of your collar with plenty of medicated powder. Most medicated powders have a cooling sensation. The powder will keep your skin dry and free of irritating sweat. The powder will also act as a soothing buffer between your collar and your delicate skin. In the evening when the shirt comes off try applying a dab of either over-the-counter cortisone cream, aloe vera gel, or a moisturizer with chamomile to the area. The anti-inflammatory nature of these products will soothe the problem area. If there are other areas of your body that have the problem of chafing and irritation you can dust these areas with the medicated powder also.

Wild-Looking Eyebrows

Are your eyebrows overgrown and out of control? Take a small scissor and trim only the hairs that are long, wiry, and going every which way. To soften the eyebrow hair so they won't seem so unruly try applying a dab of shampoo to each brow the next time you wash your hair. Rub them vigorously, then rinse well.

KEEP YOUR SKIN LOOKING YOUNG

Did you know that 80 to 90 percent of aging skin is due to sun damage? Protect your skin from the sun with a sunscreen that contains an SPF of 15 or higher any time you're exposed to sunlight. (For more information see Chapter Ten, "Tanning: The Good and the Bad.")

SUM IT UP!

This chapter focused on a few specialty treatments that address problems of concern to men: shaving, callused skin, discolored nails, neck irritation, wild eyebrows, and aging skin. But valuable information on caring for male skin can be found throughout the book. Men and women both share the same skin-care complaints and concerns; they both must deal with dryness, oiliness, blackheads, wrinkles, and blemished skin. These conditions can be kept under control if you know how to care for them. The rest of the chapters will direct you to plenty of simple, inexpensive ways to achieve problem-free skin.

CHAPTER *Eight*

SEASONAL SKIN CARE

Our lives are affected by the shifts in weather—from freezing temperatures, winds, snow, hail, sleet, and rain to heat waves and dry spells. Erosion is the end result of this chain of events.

How will your skin hold up on this never-ending roller coaster? One thing is for sure: If you don't take the necessary steps to protect your skin you will be adding the words, "weathered look" to your complexion vocabulary. This is a term that describes the effects over time of the burning sun, whipping winds, and freezing temperatures. In previous eras you could judge the harshness of the winter by the condition of the skin on someone's face. What a horrible thought!

What does our skin have to do with the seasons and the weather? The skin acts as a barometer and regulator for our bodies. It helps us adjust to external environmental factors. If we get too warm we perspire to cool down our body temperature. If we get too cold we burn more energy to help maintain our 98.6 degree body temperature. Every inch of our body is covered with this valuable external protection, but unfortunately it can be damaged by the striking blows of harsh weather as the seasons come and go.

Preventing that not-so-flattering weathered look takes only a few practical common-sense adjustments in the day-to-day care of your skin. Just as you wouldn't wear a winter coat in the middle of the summer or a bathing suit in the deep freeze of January, you must change your skin products as the climate changes. This chapter will help you get a grip on how to adjust your beauty regimen with product selections that will be compatable with your skin as it makes the transitional changes with each season.

DISCOVER THREE NATURAL ENVIRONMENTAL ELEMENTS THAT COULD DESTROY YOUR SKIN

T.H.S.

Temperature, humidity, and sun (T.H.S.) all take their toll on our skin, but each skin type is influenced in a different way. Low temperatures and low humidity strip the skin of precious moisture, causing dry or mature skin to suffer the most. High temperatures and high humidity increase perspiration, which aggravates an oily or acne complexion, and possibly initiates a host of heat-related skin disturbances. Of course, all of us can suffer from irreversible cell damage if we meet the powerful, invisible UVA, UVB, and UVC rays head-on without protection. (For detailed information about the sun refer to Chapter Ten, "Tanning.")

LEARN HOW TO DEAL WITH COLD WEATHER AND YOUR SKIN

How Do Low Humidity and Cold Temperatures Affect Dry or Mature Skin?

The surrounding air rapidly pulls moisture from your skin by means of evaporation.

Dry, mature, or sensitive skin complexions suffer the most in this type of weather because it doesn't take much to throw these delicate skin types off balance. Dry or mature skin types are lacking moisture to begin with; then along come the harsh winter months, which make matters worse by depleting the skin of what little moisture it has. Sensitive skin is such a volatile type of complexion that it doesn't do well at all with the extreme cold temperatures; skin may become red and irritated with the first cold blast.

How Do Low Humidity and Temperatures Affect Oily or Acne Skin?

Oily skin complexions rejoice with the onset of cool weather because this means a reduction of excess oil. Cold weather decreases the amount of perspiration flow to the surface of the skin. Perspiration is what makes an oily complexion more intense in the summer. In severe cold weather even an oily skin type can feel a little tight and dry.

The oil on the surface acts as a protective barrier that helps to hold moisture on the surface of the skin.

What it all boils down to is *moisture* and our ability to hold it on the surface of our skin. It is as simple as that. You can regulate, through internal and external means, the fluctuation of moisture your skin experiences during the cold months. Here are a few practical hints on how to preserve your skin's moisture.

PRACTICAL COLD WEATHER SUGGESTIONS

Internal Methods to Preserve Moisture

- Reduce intake of diuretics such as coffee and tea.
- Increase the amount of water you drink (this doesn't include soda). The American Academy of Nutrition recommends eight, 8-ounce glasses of water a day.
- Eat plenty of fresh fruit and vegetables; they contain natural vitamin-rich moisture.

External Methods to Preserve Moisture

- Gloves, hats, and scarves please! Don't let that cold wind whip at your skin.
- If your skin feels dry, select water-based products that are a little richer in consistency (they contain more natural oils). The

heavier types of moisturizers worn during the day will supply a line of first defense against the moisture-robbing cold temperatures.

- If you use soap make sure you rinse extremely well because soap residue can cause dryness and irritation.
- Extreme dry-skin sufferers should wash their face only once a day. Use your cleanser in the evening to remove your make-up, then apply your toner and night creme. In the morning gently wipe skin with your nonalcohol-based toner, then apply a rich moisturizer.

HOT WEATHER—FOUR EASY WAYS TO KEEP YOUR SKIN COOL AND DRY

Warm weather has the opposite effect on the skin because increased temperatures stimulate the sweat glands that help to regulate the heat. The dry-skin type and the oily-skin type each react quite differently to the environmental stresses of the summer months. Dry and mature skin types respond favorably to the warmth and humidity, whereas the oily- and acne-skin types become aggravated with the high temperatures and humidity because they stimulate the sweat and oil glands. (Almost all individuals will respond in a negative manner if the skin continues to be warm and moist with perspiration for any length of time, without relief.) Eczema and acne are aggravated by warm, moist skin. In many cases rashes and fungus infections can also develop under these conditions. Prickly heat is another warm weather problem. This condition occurs when the sweat gland ducts become blocked and the sweat cannot reach the surface of the skin, resulting in inflammation. Prickly heat looks like small blisters about the size of a pinhead.

The skin can adjust to many environmental stresses, but as you can see, a whole host of skin disturbances can take place when the skin is warm and moist for a prolonged period of time.

Here are a few helpful suggestions to help you defend yourself from these warm weather nuisances:

1. Wear loose-fitting clothes made from natural fibers.

2. Shower frequently to remove perspiration and cool off your body temperature.
3. Dust yourself with plain or medicated powder.
4. Sprinkle powder in your footwear.

THE "FOUR SEASONS" SURVIVAL GUIDE FOR YOUR SKIN

Winter, spring, summer and autumn—what do they all have in common? The answer is change. Our skin is constantly changing from season to season, making it seem as if our complexion is always in a state of transition. This is because our skin is an adaptive organ. It has developed a keen awareness in order to survive in a healthy condition. But as our skin changes so must our care. This doesn't mean throwing out all your products every few months; it means making a simple adjustment or two. This section will teach you how your skin type is influenced by each season and how you can take the necessary steps to protect your skin.

OILY AND ACNE SKIN—NO-FAIL WAYS TO PROTECT YOUR SKIN YEAR-ROUND

Winter (best season for oily skin)

This is probably the one time of year that you feel in control of your oily skin, but there are always exceptions. The oily condition seems to lessen a little with the cold weather because you perspire less in the winter. The harshness of the winter can even cause an oily or acne complexion to get a little tight and possibly experience some flakiness.

Seasonal Solutions: Maintenance Even an oily skin needs special care in the winter. You may have to switch your cleanser from the oil-free gel you used in the summer to a lightweight, water-based lotion or foaming creme cleanser. If you notice that your skin still feels a little tight after cleansing, you should wear a moisturizer.

Remember even an oily skin can become dehydrated during the cold months if it is neglected. A lightweight gel moisturizer or a hydrating fluid (both should be oil-free if you are prone to blemishes and blackheads) should do the trick for both day and night. And don't forget to use your facial scrub or an AHA (alpha hydroxy acid) product; it will help keep your skin smooth and free from unwanted dead skin cell buildup.

Spring

As the temperature slowly rises so do the amount of surface oils on your skin. Excess shine may develop. Even though your oily skin is somewhat under control, pre-summer preparation and care is vital if you want to control how your skin will react during the summer months.

Seasonal Solutions: Conditioning You should focus on proper cleansing and dead skin cell removal so you can avoid the buildup of oils. But don't overdo it. Morning and evening cleanings with a water-based cleansing lotion or an oil-free gel cleanser is fine. Facial scrubs should be used no more than twice a week. (Do not use them at all if you have acne skin.) If you don't usually use a clay masque, this is the time when you should begin, because it will help to temporarily absorb any excess oils. (Use twice a week and leave on for 10 to 15 minutes.)

Summer (the worst season for oily skin)

The heat of the summer causes increased perspiration. The perspiration acts as a vehicle to distribute your skin's oil all over your face, making your skin feel and look more shiny during the hot, humid months of summer. If you have an acne condition this is the time it usually flares up and becomes a nuisance.

Seasonal Solutions: Protect This is the time to pay serious attention to your skin. If you are suffering with an uncontrollable amount of excess oil it may be necessary to switch your cleanser and moisturizer to an oil-free kind. Foaming gel cleansers and gel moisturizers seem to work well in the summer. A nonalcohol-based astringent that uses botanicals has degreasing properties so it works wonders in the summer. Increase your clay masque usage from two to three times a week if your skin is extra oily. Selecting the wrong foundation in the summer can be disastrous for your skin. If you are using a liquid type it is best to switch to a matte foundation because it will absorb the excess oils.

Autumn

The temperatures are lower and so is the level of oil. Your skin is just beginning to respond in a favorable way. But now, as the crisis of the summer months passes, the skin needs a little help in the recovery process.

Seasonal Solutions: Recondition You may see the residual effects of the excess oils of summer. Enlarged pores may be prevalent at this time, causing your complexion to look a little coarser in texture. There is nothing that can permanently make your pores smaller in size, but you might try a cleanser and moisturizer with alpha hydroxy acids. The AHAs in the product will help remove the buildup of dead skin cells, helping to create a slightly smoother surface. If you like the cleanser and moisturizer you're using now and don't want to switch products then try a facial scrub. The scrub will also remove dead skin cells. Moisturizing (oil-free type of products) your skin at this time is important; you do not want your skin to become dehydrated before the cold weather hits. If you're using a clay masque, decrease the usage to once a week as the temperature gets cooler.

Seasonal Timetable for Oily or Acne Skin

All Year Round Sunscreen should not be reserved only for the summer. An oil-free sunscreen with at least an SPF of 15 should be used all year long.

Winter Adjust your skin-care program by switching your oil-free cleanser and moisturizer to a water-based lotion. The oil-free type may be too drying for your skin at this time of year.

Spring Focus on deep cleansing and removal of dead skin cells to help prepare your skin for the summer months. Use a natural-bristle complexion brush to aid you in the cleansing process.

Summer Oil-free products during this time are a must if you suffer from excessive oiliness. Proper cleansing is always important but is especially so in the summer. Try cleansing your face twice in the evening because the extra oils in the summer make it very difficult to remove make-up. Clay masque treatments two to three times a week will help absorb excess oils.

Autumn It's important to make sure your skin is properly hydrated at this time, so use a lightweight, water-based moisturizer. Exfoliating products will help to create a smoother complexion. Also, reduce the use of your clay masque to once a week.

DRY OR MATURE SKIN—WAYS YOU CAN SHIELD YOUR SKIN IN ALL SEASONS

Winter (worst season for dry or mature skin)

Freezing temperatures and reduced humidity make the cold months an extremely unfriendly environment for any skin type but especially so for dry and mature skin. This type of harsh atmosphere robs the skin of precious moisture, creating a situation that makes the skin susceptible to irritation, chapping, and extreme dryness. Minor changes in your daily routine must be taken to avoid severe problems.

Seasonal Solutions: Protection Concentrate on extra moisturizing. Giving your skin the added protection it needs may be as simple as switching to richer products that contain more emollients. Cleansers, moisturizers, and night cremes with a higher oil content will help create a barrier that will hold moisture to the skin. The extra oils in the products help slow down the evaporation of water from the skin.

Night cremes and pure dry oils (squalane, almond, or macadamia nut oil) can be a salvation during extreme dry-skin weather conditions. As you sleep with these skin-softening products on your skin, you will be preparing your skin for the next day. So don't skip a night.

If you're experiencing chapped lips it may be necessary to apply an over-the-counter antibiotic ointment to your lips. It will help heal the problem.

Lip balms and rich eye cremes can help protect these two delicate areas.

Spring

Spring is in the air as moderate temperatures and increased humidity become a welcome relief to dry and mature skin. At this time your skin may still have the telltale signs of the harsh effects of the winter.

Seasonal Solutions: Reconditioning Moisturizing dry skin is always important, but you should also focus on reducing the buildup of dead skin cells by using either facial scrubs or an alpha hydroxy acid product. Intensive serum concentrates of herbal fluids or oils (available in ampule, capsule, or bottle form) can help condition a parched complexion. This type of product works well under night cremes.

Summer (best season for dry and mature skin)

Warm temperatures and added humidity gently blanket your skin with precious moisture. Dry skin types respond favorably to the welcome warmth of the season. Smart maintenance can make your skin have a healthy appearance.

Seasonal Solution: Maintenance You may have to retire those rich products and save them in a cool, dry place until winter. It may be necessary to switch your cleanser, moisturizer, and night creme to a lighter, water-based product. Take special care in the cleansing process. This may be the only season that a dry or mature skin can cleanse twice a day. And don't forget to rinse well. A moisturizing masque should be used only once a week.

Autumn

Dry or mature skin beware: It is almost that time of year that strips your skin of moisture. The key emphasis this season is on conditioning. If your skin is in the best possible condition when winter hits you won't have as many problems.

Seasonal Solutions: Therapeutic Conditioning Bathe your skin in much needed moisture because by this time of year your skin is beginning to show the first signs of extra dryness. Be good to your skin by treating it with a creamy, nondrying type of masque twice a week. Before applying the masque slough off dead skin cells with a facial scrub. A rich eye product and lip balm can condition the eye area before it becomes dry. Apply this product morning and night.

Seasonal Timetable for Dry or Mature Complexions

All Year Round Sunscreens with an SPF of 15 or higher should be used all year long.

Winter Use a rich cleanser, moisturizer, and night creme. Don't use any type of textured washcloth or textured sponge because they are too rough to use when your skin is in this extra dry state. Switch to a smooth sponge or chamois type of cloth. (You can find these cleansing accessories in most salon, spa, and bath shops.)

Spring Recondition your skin with the use of a facial scrub or alpha hydroxy acid product accompanied with an intense oil or serum (botanical) concentrate. A soft-bristle complexion brush gives a new dimension to the cleansing routine. Be extra gentle; don't use too much pressure on the skin.

Summer Switch to lighter, water-based skin-care products. Too much oil in a product at this time may be overwhelming to your skin. Textured cleansing sponges are a great cleansing tool because they help improve circulation.

Autumn Alpha hydroxy acid products can be used at this time to keep the skin looking fresh and free from an accumulation of dead skin cells.

Skin Condition Forecast

This skin condition forecast will alert you to what you can expect at different temperatures so you can take the necessary precautions.

90-100°

- oily complexions become noticeably shinier due to the increased persperation.

80°

- blemish flare-up due to the heat and perspiration
- prickly heat
- fungus conditions
- rashes

60-70°

- excellent temperatures for the skin

50°

- start to notice the beginning of dryer skin

40°

- dryness

30°

- chapped skin

20°

- scaly, flaky skin, overexposure could cause frostbite

10°

- severe dryness, overexposure could cause frostbite

0°

- irritated, cracked skin, overexposure could cause frostbite

SOOTHING RECOVERY TREATMENTS FOR EXTREME WEATHER SKIN PROBLEMS

Extraordinary measures may be needed to help reverse the effects from the cold blasts of winter and the blistering heat of summer. The next three beauty prescriptions call upon special techniques plus herb, floral, and fruit essences to help rescue you from extreme weather conditions. After using these recovery treatments you will begin to feel refreshed and alive again.

The Ultimate Hand Reconditioning Remedy for Winter Weather

Are your hands beginning to look as red as a lobster? Are they cracked and irritated and burned? Here's an intensive conditioning glove treatment that will help you survive the harsh effects of low temperatures and low humidity.

Supplies

- facial cleanser (Do not cleanse your hands with soap when they are irritated. Use your facial cleanser as long as it is not an oil-free or medicated type for acne.) An oatmeal-based soap (most pharmacies have this product) is an excellent alternative for cleansing the hands and will help to soothe irritation.
- over-the-counter antibiotic ointment or A&D Ointment (you can find these items in any pharmacy)
- oil-based hand creme (the kind that leaves a film on your skin) or tube of pure lanolin (call your pharmacy; they may have to order it for you)
- petroleum jelly or massage creme
- disposable latex or vinyl gloves and cotton gloves (found in pharmacy)

Step One: Cleanse And Medicate. Wash hands with facial cleanser and rinse well. While your skin is still moist apply the over-the-counter antibiotic ointment to irritated and cracked areas.

Step Two: Recondition and Therapeutic Covering (1) Apply the oil-based hand creme or lanolin to your hands and massage onto skin. If you see a film of product on your skin you know you have applied the correct amount. (2) Next, apply a thick coat of petroleum jelly or massage creme over both hands. The function of this product is to lie on the surface of the skin and prevent the evaporation of any moisture from your hand creme.

Step Three: Therapeutic Covering (1) Place your hands into the cotton gloves. You may have to wipe off any overflow of petroleum jelly from the outside of the gloves. (2) Once all is clean, place your hands into a pair of disposable latex gloves. Keep this treatment on for a couple of hours (do your housework, catch up on reading, or watch your favorite TV show). (3) Remove the gloves and any excess petroleum jelly or creme that is left on your skin. Your skin should feel smooth and there should be much less irritation.

Note: For an overnight treatment, use only the cotton gloves. The A&D Ointment (formulated for diaper rash) works great as an overnight treatment. Massage generously on hands, especially the top and the knuckles and put on the cotton gloves. In the morning your hands will look like new.

The Two-Minute Forestral Leg Energizer for Hot Weather (also excellent for tired legs year round)

Do your legs feel like lead as you trudge through the hot summer months? Can't take another step? Here's a little treat that will help you rescue your fatigued, overheated legs. Capture the cooling and energizing essences of the forest and let woody pine, floral lavender, and mentholated peppermint refresh you immediately.
Supplies:

- body lotion (any kind will do)
- pine, lavender, and peppermint essential oils (three individual oils)

Step One: Preparation Add a drop of each of the essential oils to a portion of body lotion like this:

- Cup your hand and pour a portion of body lotion into your hand.
- Add the 3 drops of essential oils.
- Mix the product by bringing both your hands together to combine the lotion and oils.

This is a very unscientific method of mixing but it's easy. If you want to mix the products in a small disposable cup or kitchen bowl that's fine too.

Step Two: Energizing Treatment Apply the body lotion that has been mixed with the essential oils to your feet and legs. Begin at your feet and work your way up, finishing at your thighs. To make this application more than just slapping lotion on your legs, massage it into your skin concentrating on areas of distress such as your toes, the arch of both feet, ankles, and the backs of your legs.

Step Three: Be Good to Yourself Sit back, place a pillow under your feet, and have a cup of soothing herbal tea. Rest for five minutes.

Mint Julep Bath Escape for Overheated Nerves

Summer heat can zap every ounce of energy from you. Replenishing your energy and soothing your overheated, frazzled nerves can be as simple as bathing in the refreshing essences of mint and orange blossom essential oils. A dip in fragrant minty and fruity waters can transform you to a relaxed state in just minutes. You will feel as fresh as spring.

Supplies:

- peppermint essential oils
- orange blossom essential oils
- body lotion
- pre-chilled washcloth or pre-filled eye masque to use as eye compress

Step One: Preparation If you are using a washcloth as the eye compress, moisten it with water and wring out the excess, then place it into a plastic bag and put it in the refrigerator for a few minutes to chill the cloth. While your bath is running add 6 to 7 drops each of peppermint and orange blossom essential oil. Your bath water should not be too hot; the temperature should be slightly warmer than tepid.

Step Two: Refreshing Treatment Before entering the tub apply one drop of peppermint essential oil that has been mixed with 2 drops of unscented oil (example jojoba oil) to each of your temples. Step into your bath and apply the chilled eye compress. Keeping your eyes closed is an important part of this treatment because it helps to reduce stress. Now all you have to do is relax for 15 to 20 minutes.

Step Three: Conditioning Step out of the bath and pat your skin dry. Then apply your favorite body lotion.

Tips to Enhance the Mint Julep Treatment

- Play soothing music while you're in the tub.
- Light a candle or two and shut off the lights.
- Add a drop of peppermint oil to a portion of your body lotion before it is applied.
- If you don't want to use an eye compress light a floating candle and place it in the tub with you. Focusing on the flame will help you forget the stresses of the day.
- After the bath, sip your favorite chilled juice or mineral water in a tall frosty glass.

AN ALL-WEATHER ALERT BULLETIN THAT COULD SAVE YOUR SKIN

Precautions and Helpful Hints for Outdoor Activities

Outdoor activities place us in direct contact with the elements. Whether you're outdoors for fun or work, you need to become more aware of the environment and to take a few simple steps to help you prevent weather-related skin disturbances from occurring.

Skin Tip for Tennis, Walking, Jogging, Running, and Rollerskating

- Wear a sunscreen with at least a 15 SPF. And don't forget to reapply as needed.
- Wear sunglasses.
- Sprinkle powder in your footwear to help absorb perspiration. This will help prevent fungus infections.
- Before dressing apply a light application of dusting powder around your waist (where the elastic rubs the skin) and torso area. This will help prevent prickly heat, which is caused by elevated temperatures and moisture.
- Shower immediately after any of these activities because excessive perspiration can cause a skin rash.
- Drink plenty of water before and after each activity.

Three Skin Tips for Swimming

- Do not shave or wax your legs, bikini line, underarms, or face the same day you intend to swim in either a chlorinated pool or the ocean. The chlorine or salt can cause a rashlike irritation (folliculitis) to your hair follicle. Plan your hair removal ahead of time.
- Shower immediately after swimming in a chlorinated pool or in salt water. These two substances can irritate and dry the skin if not removed. Moisturize your skin with a body lotion after swimming.
- Wear the strongest sunscreen you can find. When swimming outdoors the potency of the UV rays is increased because of the reflection of the water. Reapply your sunscreen frequently.

Four Skin Tips for Gardening

- Wear sunscreen with at least an SPF of 15.
- Wear a wide-brim hat.
- Use gloves at all times if you don't want to destroy your hands. Apply a hand and cuticle creme before applying the gloves. To help prevent your nails from breaking or getting stained with dirt here is a little tip: Take a bar of soap and dig your nails into the bar until you have enough soap wedged under each nail to act as a cushion. Then place your hands into the gloves. After

gardening take a nail brush and scrub gently to remove the soap. If you don't like the bulky feel of gardening gloves try wearing latex examination gloves. They cling to the skin and won't interfere with your dexterity. You can find these gloves in a pharmacy or medical-supply store.

- Protect your knees from getting callused. Cut the feet off a pair of old white tube socks. Apply a rich body lotion over your knees, then apply petroleum jelly over the creme. Slip into the cut tube socks and cover your knees; then slip into your pants. This will be a conditioning treatment and when you kneel it will help prevent stains and calluses from forming.

SUM IT UP!

Understanding the seasonal needs of your skin is a preventive way to protect your skin from seasonal problems or, even worse, permanent skin damage. Don't forget to safeguard your skin from the many natural environmental elements that await you, and follow the seasonal transition-cycle information in this chapter so you will know how to adjust your skin-care regimen to the weather. A heightened awareness and a keen sensitivity to the hazards of the ever-changing climate can help you preserve the youthfulness of your complexion.

CHAPTER *Nine*

TIMELESS BEAUTY

UNDERSTANDING THE DYNAMICS OF CARING FOR MATURE SKIN

A bottle of wine, works of art, and fine antiques. What do these luxurious items have in common? They all improve with age—if they are properly protected from the environment. The same is true of your skin, which accumulates most of its damage from environmental abuse and physical traumas. Aging is not a disease, but a natural process. It can affect the skin in a slow, subtle manner or very rapidly, depending on whether you abuse your skin or protect it. If you abuse it, it's not likely to improve with age and you may end up unhappy with your appearance and with a bad case of lowered self-esteem.

If you want to preserve and improve the quality of your complexion, minimize imperfections, and keep your skin healthy-looking throughout your life, you'll be happy to learn that it isn't difficult. Stop smoking. Eat a balanced diet. Keep your skin clean and free of dirt and oils, and don't suntan. Simply follow these guidelines and you're more than halfway to achieving timeless beauty.

This chapter addresses the highly emotional subject of aging. It examines how aging affects the skin and how these effects can be minimized or avoided altogether. As you read, you'll learn about the physiological changes that occur in your twenties, thirties, forties, fifties, and sixties. Armed with this information, you'll discover how to achieve timeless beauty at any life stage by understanding your skin's special needs. As you've already discovered, you don't need cosmetic surgery to maintain and improve your complexion.

With the first sign of aging, we begin scrutinizing our skin. Usually, the first thing we notice is that our eyes look a little tired or that we have a hint of fine lines just underneath the surface of our skin. If we overscrutinize, it can seem as though new imperfections appear every day. Too many bad skin days and we start seeking fountain-of-youth remedies, treatments, and prescriptions. But fountain-of-youth promises aren't the answer: common sense, coupled with science, is. The first rule of common sense says that a happy and relaxed mind is reflected in beautiful skin.

YOU'RE AS YOUNG AS YOUR ATTITUDE

Holding on to youthfulness means more than applying skin creme. If you embrace each stage of life passionately and live abundantly, you will be young forever. Staying young also depends on your frame of mind—your attitude. If you have a youthful, energetic attitude, you will portray a youthful image. If you have a sad or negative attitude, you will look old before your time. My grandmother, Mildred Parentini, who lived to be 100, embraced life with a youthful exuberance. When I'd ask her how she felt she'd reply, "In my heart, I feel like I'm sixteen years old." She always told me, "It's better to be like a willow tree than an oak tree in a storm, because the willow will bend and survive the storm; the oak tree will break under the pressure of the wind." This was my grandmother's way of saying that if you can reduce your day-to-day stress by being flexible, your life will be much more enjoyable. Stress has a direct effect on your health and is ultimately reflected in your skin. Have you ever seen someone and immediately thought, "She had a hard life"? Chances are, she had a stressful life and dealt with that stress by turning to cigarettes, alcohol, or drugs.

An old wives' tale says that if you make a face too often, it will freeze in place. There is a certain truth to this. If you constantly frown, furrows in your forehead will deepen. While those furrows might be genetically encoded, you can minimize or maximize this predisposition by living happily. No one can be joyous all the time, but how you deal with sorrow matters tremendously. To lessen sadness and stress, practice deep breathing and relaxation techniques. Be honest about how you're feeling; don't try to repress emotions or deny that you're feeling stressful. Remind yourself what's worth getting upset over and what isn't. And if problems seem overwhelming, never be afraid to seek help. It's well documented that stress can bring on headaches, weaken the body's immune system, and even interfere with the normal function of organs, such as the heart. It's no wonder that stress shows up in your skin too.

VILLAINS THAT COULD AGE YOUR SKIN BEFORE ITS TIME

Philosophers say you begin to age the moment you're born; most physicians say that the tell-tale signs of maturing usually begin to appear around age 30. This figure is not written in stone; you can protect your skin and care for it in a manner that staves off aging, just as you can hasten premature aging. I've seen people in their late twenties whose abusive habits have already begun to damage their skin, and I've seen individuals in their sixties who have the complexion of a forty year old.

What kind of abuse ages the skin before its time? Poor nutrition, alcohol, and drug intake, smoking, sun exposure, excessive stress, chronic illness, lack of exercise, and a negative attitude. You never hear anyone say, "I can't wait until I have wrinkles," but every time you get either a tan or a sunburn, smoke excessively, eat poorly, exacerbate stress, go a week without exercise, or binge on alcohol, you're making yourself susceptible to premature aging. Another hazard that affects the health and integrity of our skin is free radicals, which also develop from a negative lifestyle. These "out of control," microscopic molecules are on a seek-and-destroy mission looking for healthy cells. Cigarette smoking, alcohol binging, fried foods, ultraviolet radiation, and air pollution all trigger the manufacture of this toxic maverick by-product. Ultimately, if these molecules damage and destroy enough healthy cells they can weaken our overall health as well as cause premature aging. If you want to preserve a youthful complexion, begin nurturing your body before it's too late. After all, there is a point of no return, when non-surgical skin care will not have much effect.

HOW LONG CAN YOU EXPECT YOUR SKIN TO LOOK GOOD?

If you are blessed with good genes and health, and if you protect your skin from the sun, you can expect to have almost the same skin quality you had in your thirties when you reach your sixties. Ninety percent of the skin's aging is due to environmental causes, with unprotected sun exposure being first on the list. It is important to distinguish between the two different forms of aging. One is caused by sun exposure and the other is chronological aging.

Wrinkles, leathery-looking skin, and frecklelike blotches and age spots are primarily caused by years of unprotected sun exposure. If your parents did not protect you with a sunscreen when you were a child or if you suntanned throughout your teens, you might see the consequences as early as age 20.

Signs of chronological aging appear later. Changes in facial contours, increased dryness and new patterns of hair growth are caused by the passage of time. Such physical and hormonal changes begin to become evident when you're in your late thirties or early forties.

ONLY TIME WILL TELL—THE AGING CYCLE

Aging affects the natural function of cell repair, cell production, and cellular turnover. All three of these vital skin functions slow down as you get older. The breakdown of the collagen and elastin proteins doesn't occur overnight; it is a slow process. Of course, if sun damage triggers the premature aging process, a 40-, 30-, or even a 20-year-old stratum corneum could metamorphose and become uneven in color. This unevenness is a prelude to age spots, to the transformation of fine lines into deep wrinkles, and to a rough and sallow skin texture.

Predicting what your skin is going to look like 10, 20, or even 30 years from now is difficult. No one knows when the first fine line, wrinkle, sag, or age spot will appear. However, there are many preventive steps, skin-care treatments, and medical options you can seek out that will help you invest in the future of your skin so that you can keep your complexion glowing for years to come.

The following information will help you care for your skin's special needs as you traverse each of life's major stages.

NO-NONSENSE STEPS YOU CAN TAKE TO HAVE PERFECT SKIN IN YOUR TWENTIES

- Eighty percent of your lifetime's worth of sun damage has occurred before you reach the age of 18. By the time you're 20, it's too late to prevent most of it if you haven't been using a sun protector or a sunblock. However, good skin-care habits that are established now will pay off in years to come.
- Your skin's collagen proteins, which begin to decrease at a rate of approximately 1 to 2 percent each year after the age of 20, help keep the skin toned and plump.
- It's rare to see wrinkles at this point in your life, but keep in mind that every time you expose your skin to the sun without using a sunscreen or a sunblock, you are causing your skin to age before its time.
- You may experience some oiliness, especially in the T-zone, and occasional flare-ups of blemishes or acne.

Nonmedical Options—Simple Skin Care You Can Do at Home

Now is the time to get serious about protecting your skin. One of the most inexpensive, over-the-counter, age-fighting products is a maximum-strength sunscreen with an SPF of 15 or higher. Apply it lavishly any time you will be in the sun or outdoors. (Even on cloudy days, the sun's harmful rays reach your skin.)

If you're good to your skin in your twenties, you'll hold on to your youthful glow into your thirties, forties, and even your fifties. Don't take your youthful complexion for granted; avoid sun exposure and tanning beds. Use a self-tanning product instead (see Chapter Ten for more details).

How a Dermatologist Can Correct Skin Problems In Your Twenties

Medical-strength peels, such as glycolic acid peels, can be performed when you're as young as 20. (Peels dissolve the top layer of skin, making the skin look smoother.) In some cases, dermatologists prescribe Retin-A to be used in the evening and a glycolic acid treatment to be used in the morning as a dual treatment for sun-damaged skin.

Retin A should be used with great care and only according to a doctor's instructions. Do not combine a glycolic treatment with Retin-A without telling your physician that you are doing so and asking for combination usage instructions. Take a break from one or both when the physician tells you to; don't continue using them in the hope you'll see even greater improvement. Skin needs a rest from most over-the-counter products; it definitely needs a break from prescription-strength drugs.

SKIN SENSE— PREVENTIVE STEPS TO HAVE GREAT-LOOKING SKIN IN YOUR THIRTIES

- Everyone ages at different rates, based on the amount of sun exposure you've sustained, your genetic makeup, your overall health, and other influences, such as excessive smoking and alcohol intake. But in your thirties your skin will probably begin to show its first sign of aging.
- Oil production from the sebaceous gland begins to decrease as you mature. This causes the skin to become dry.
- In your thirties, your skin type is likely to change slightly. An oily skin type might become more normalized; a normal skin type will begin to feel a little dryer. A dry skin type will suffer the most because the aging process exacerbates dryness.
- Stress, oral contraceptives, or pregnancy can trigger adult acne. It is important to be aware of changes in your skin type so you can make the necessary adjustments in your day-to-day skin-care routine.

- The inner structure that supports your skin will begin to show its first signs of weakness. Collagen production decreases and your elastin fibers become less pliable, so your skin becomes less flexible.
- Elasticity and tone have a direct effect on your facial muscles. A lifetime of making natural movements, such as squinting, smiling, or frowning, begins to map out your complexion. Hints of crow's feet, frown lines, or laugh lines may begin to surface.
- The redistribution and loss of fat in the subcutaneous level of the skin causes it to begin to sag.

Learn How to Nurture Your Skin at Home

Take stronger steps to prevent accumulating any more sun damage. Replace your day moisturizer with one that contains a sunscreen with an SPF of 15 or higher. Recognize that changes are taking place in your skin and address those changes by adjusting your skin-care routine and/or skin-care products.

If your skin shows signs of dryness, stop using the cleanser and moisturizer you used in your twenties because they may no longer be adequate. Because your skin has decreased its oil production, you may need to use products with more emollients in them to help replace the lost oil. If you're afraid that these richer products will feel greasy, select ones that are water-based. With today's sophisticated skin-care technology, most emollient-laden products are light to the touch.

Skin Makeover! Revolutionary Ways a Dermatologist Can Freshen Your Complexion in Your Thirties

If you have sun-damaged skin, a physician may suggest that you begin repairing it by combining peels with Retin-A usage. Options in peels include medical-strength glycolic acid peels or superficial chemical peels, such as a trichloracetic acid peel, a Jessner's Solution peel, a salicylic acid peel, or a solid carbon dioxide peel.

A dermatologist can tell you if combining peels and Retin-A usage will revive your complexion, improve your skin tone, or minimize fine lines and enlarged pores. In many cases it's possible. Remember, any time you use these treatments alone or in combination, sun avoidance is absolutely essential, as is following your dermatologist's usage instructions for Retin-A.

BE YOUR SKIN'S BEST FRIEND—IMPORTANT FACTS THAT WILL HELP YOU SLOW THE AGING PROCESS IN YOUR FORTIES

- Whichever forms of aging you noticed in your thirties will become more pronounced in your forties. You'll also see a few new surface changes. The aging process takes place slowly if your skin is undamaged, but if you abused your complexion with unprotected sun exposure, your aging will progress at a much faster rate.
- Changes you might notice include creases in your forehead area, crow's feet around the outer corners of your eyes, a fine, wrinkled texture (crepiness) to your eyelid, fine lines from frowning, puffiness under your eyes, and a feathering of fine lines around your lip line. At first, these symptoms will be extremely faint and appear to be below the skin's surface, then they gradually will become more pronounced.

Discover What You Can Do to Help Your Skin Stay in Tip-Top Shape

If dryness is a problem, switching from water-based gel products to skin-care treatments with a creamy consistency may be necessary. Also, consider products that contain alpha hydroxy acids (AHAs). You might also want to add new products to both your morning and evening repertoires, such as eye creams, lip balms, and night cremes. Experiment with what works for you, suits your budget, and accommodates your lifestyle. Often, a single product can act as an overall moisturizer for face, hands, and body. Give moisturizers a boost by spritzing your face with water whenever practical.

If you are still not satisfied with the feel and texture of your skin, try using a serum, which can be worn under your day moisturizer or night creme. Serums are highly concentrated with active ingredients; therefore, a small amount goes a long way. When you address your skin's need for moisture in this manner, your complexion will appear fresher because the water and emollients in the products will temporarily plump up the stratum corneum. Also, focus on removing dead skin cells by exfoliating with a mild facial scrub or by using a product that contains AHAs. Once a week is ample; don't overexfoliate.

If you have not yet taken preventive steps to avoid all sun exposure, do so. Use a sunscreen with an SPF of 15 or higher every day. Keep in mind that it takes a sunscreen about half an hour to be absorbed into your skin. Wait at least that long after applying it before going outdoors.

Banish Sun-Damaged and Premature-Aged Skin in Your Forties

Continue with whichever type of superficial skin peels you used in your thirties, or consider starting them. You may also want to explore laser treatments to repair actinic keratoses and age spots caused by accumulated sun damage.

Plumping up the skin with fillers such as collagen and fat transplants is also an option that will help keep your complexion youthful. However, these can become very expensive, since they must be repeated on a regular basis—sometimes yearly. (These are discussed in greater depth in Chapter Twelve.)

INEXPENSIVE STEPS THAT WILL PRESERVE YOUR YOUTHFULNESS IN YOUR FIFTIES

- During this decade, gravity and menopause have a profound effect on the skin. Fluctuations in hormonal levels can trigger a temporary case of adult acne, which will abate after menopause.
- Gravity, the rapid decrease in collagen production, and elastic rigidity quickly cause your skin to lose its tone. Your complex-

ion can take on a tired, drawn appearance, which may be particularly evident around the eyes and jawline. Eyelids will droop; the area under the eyes may become puffy, and the jawline might sag.

- Have you ever heard someone say that the older you get, the larger your nose and ears become? These features appear to grow only because of the effect that gravity has on the cartilage. The cartilage acts as a support for the skin, much like a beam in a wall. If the beam begins to droop, so does the wall. As cartilage droops, so does your skin. When this occurs, your ears and nose appear longer.
- Your skin will continue to become dryer, and its texture may become rough, depending on how much sun damage you've accumulated.

Dynamic Steps that Will Keep Your Skin Youthful in Your Fifties

By the time you reach your fifties, your skin may have become more sensitive because of dryness. If this is the case, switch from lighter, water-based products to thicker, richer ones. You may even want to try an oil-based cleanser, so that your skin does not dry out during the cleansing process. Moisturizing is crucial if you want to maintain the integrity of the skin's surface. Dehydration makes your skin more rigid and less pliable; it also accentuates fine lines and wrinkles.

Look for day moisturizers and night creams that are bolstered with skin-softening, active ingredients, such as humectants and emollients. Humectants help hold moisture in the skin; emollients, which act like a barrier, slow the evaporation of moisture from the surface of the skin. If you haven't started to use products that contain AHAs, now is a good time to start. These products will help remove unwanted, dead skin cells, which if allowed to accumulate will cause your skin to look dull, rough, and flaky.

There's no reason to pay a fortune for skin-care products; often, less expensive products are more effective than costly ones because expensive products include the price of fancy packaging and corporate advertising. Check past issues of magazines such as

Consumer Reports, which test products, to help you choose one that is effective and suits your budget. If you haven't been using a sunscreen with an SPF of 15 or higher on a daily basis, start doing so.

Dermatologic Options—Learn How a Dermatologist Can Help Erase Fine Lines, Wrinkles, and Uneven Color in Your Fifties

During your fifties, a deeper chemical peel, called a phenol peel, may be necessary to soften the uneven skin tones, age spots, and wrinkles that are caused by accumulated sun damage. Retin-A may be prescribed as a part of your regular skin-care routine. Remember, you should build up tolerance to Retin-A slowly. If you're already using it, your dermatologist may switch you from the creme version to the more effective gel formulation.

Skin Rejuvenation! Discover Which Cosmetic Surgical Procedures Can Create a More Youthful Complexion Puffiness under the eyes and a loose, crepy skin on the upper eyelids can create a tired, older appearance. These undesirable changes can be modified with an eye lift (bleparoplasty). Another option to investigate is called rhytidectomy, or a face lift. During a face lift, the muscles and sagging tissue are tightened, excess fat and skin are removed, and any fat that is creating a double chin is eliminated, so that the face has a more youthful contour. (These options are discussed in greater depth in Chapter Twelve.)

IT'S NOT NICE TO FOOL MOTHER NATURE—DYNAMIC WAYS THAT WILL HELP RENEW YOUR COMPLEXION IN YOUR SIXTIES

- Bone loss, loss of teeth, and redistribution or loss of fat in the subcutaneous level of the skin play tremendous roles in the three-dimensional aspect of your facial structure. We tend to concentrate on the changes that occur at the skin's surface, but there are many changes that occur at the skeletal level. These changes affect the draping of your skin, particularly on the lower half of the face.

- Problems you had in previous decades become more pronounced in your sixties. These might include loss of skin tone, wrinkles, crow's feet, frown lines, age spots, smile lines, thinning lips, and sallowness.

Nonmedical Options

Use mild, nonaggressive skin-care products that contain no alcohol or potentially irritating artificial fragrances. Avoid harsh facial scrubs that contain large grains; use an AHA-containing product or a scrub with microscopic grains instead.

If your skin shows signs of excessive dryness, use oil-based products instead of water-based ones. Oil-based products will help protect and soften fragile skin and prevent it from losing additional moisture. At nighttime, experiment with specialty products. Ones you might try include eye creme, lip balm, or a highly concentrated serum, worn under your moisturizer or night creme. At this stage of your life, your skin produces very little natural oil and these products satisfy the skin's need for oil; however, they must be used on a daily basis to achieve and maintain results. Always wear a product containing a sunscreen with an SPF of at least 15 anytime you go outdoors.

Rx for Aging Skin! Innovative Dermatologic Procedures that Will Take Years Off Your Complexion

Deep chemical peels (TCA peels and phenol peels) in combination with laser surgery or injectable collagen or fat fillers can help to freshen your complexion and minimize surface imperfections such as wrinkles and age spots.

Supercharge Mature Skin! Cosmetic Surgical Procedures that Create a More Youthful Appearance

A full face and neck lift (rhytidectomy) and upper and lower eye lift (bleparoplasty) will help minimize the changes that are taking place in your sixties due to the redistribution of fat, loss of bone, and loss of skin tone. (These options are discussed in greater depth in Chapter Twelve.)

YOUR SKIN AFTER MENOPAUSE

Even if your skin is undamaged by the sun, it will show subtle changes after menopause. A slowdown in oil production causes the skin either to thin or thicken in certain areas. Blotchiness and dryness can occur because of fluctuating hormone levels. The skin on your body tends to age much more gracefully than facial skin because your body has been protected from the sun by clothing.

The older you get, the more vulnerable to environmental effects your skin becomes; however, sun-damaged skin loses the most elasticity and tone because of overexposure to UV rays and the underlying damage that results. After menopause, the middle layer of the skin thins out and its ability to retain water is diminished. Changes in facial contours occur because of the redistribution of fat cells and loss of fat in the lower level of the skin or the subcutaneous level.

SMOOTHING AWAY THE YEARS AT ANY LIFE STAGE

There is no quick way to turn back the clock. It may have taken twenty, thirty, forty, fifty, or sixty years for your skin to reach the condition it is in today. However, your skin is always the youngest organ of your body because it goes through a regenerative process every 28 days. So, a new skin is always just below the surface.

But what are your options for achieving a more youthful complexion? Who are the nonmedical and medical professionals who can help you when you want to enhance the quality of your skin? And what is the truth about the prescription products that claim to improve your skin's appearance? How do they really work?

The quest for anti-aging products in the United States has never been more intense. This is because the "me generation" is showing its first sign of wrinkles, and it doesn't like what it sees. With the U.S. median age at 32.9 years, the next 10 years will see a large portion of the baby boomers move into maturity. Maturing skin definitely has special needs that are fully recognized by the dermatological, cosmetic surgery, and beauty industries, which are performing valuable research on aging skin. New types of peels, improved surgical procedures, and skin-enhancing ingredients are always being introduced.

OVER-THE-COUNTER SKIN CARE THAT WILL REJUVENATE MATURE OR SUN-DAMAGED SKIN

Keep in mind when searching for products for sun-damaged and mature skin that they should have special properties. The moisturizing efficacy of any product you select is the key factor in maintaining the integrity, health, and appearance of your skin. At this point the skin has become deficient of two of the most valuable components: sebum (the skin's natural oils) and moisture. The symptoms of this excessively dry, dehydrated, and possibly sluggish condition is as follows: The skin suffers flakiness and tightness; it may look dull; skin becomes rigid and less pliable, and fine lines and wrinkles become more visible.

The part of the skin that over-the-counter moisturizing products affect, whether a cleanser, toner, or moisturizer, is the stratum corneum of the epidermis. This outermost layer of your skin is about the thickness of a piece of tape but its protective importance to our body outweighs its size. You can better understand the function of moisturizing when you understand the composition of the stratum corneum. The outermost layer of the skin consists of 20 percent lipids (cementlike material consisting of triglycerides, free fatty acids, waxes, free sterol, squalene, paraffin, and ceramides, which help hold the skin cells together and retain moisture), 40 percent water, and 40 percent protein (mostly keratin, from dead skin cells). And as we age, the skin's ability to hold moisture is compromised because of the deficiency in the cementlike substance called lipids. This valuable component of the skin has an exceptional protective role because it acts somewhat like a sealant. When a deficiency takes place in this area of the skin it lessens the skin's capacity for protection; the result is a loss of moisture and possible irritation. Mature and sun-damaged skin is not able to maintain the proper moisture level to keep it looking fresh and dewy. It needs daily assistance from you.

The stratum corneum is able to recover from extreme dryness because of its unusual composition, which is somewhat like a sponge and which makes it easy to rehydrate. If a product containing enough barrier-forming, water-impermeable ingredients (essential fatty acids) is applied to the skin, the stratum corneum will absorb five to six times its dry weight and hold this moisture to the skin. The thickness in turn will evenly increase by approximately four times its original size. This increased thickness helps to temporarily camouflage and diminish any fine lines to give you the appearance of a fresher-looking complexion.

The function of a moisturizing product is threefold: the water in the formula is absorbed by the stratum corneum, the humectant (glycerin, sodium hyaluronic acid, sorbitol, or mannitol to name a few) attracts moisture to this area, and then the emollient (essential fatty acids: linoleic acid, oleic acids, squalane, or natural plant oils) function as a sealant to help slow up the evaporation process and hold this newfound moisture to the surface of the skin. This, of course, is a temporary plumping situation, and the results will vary with each individual, from climate to climate and with the richness of the product, but the rule of thumb says you should apply a moisturizer twice a day or as needed.

If you're not quite sure which products will successfully address the needs of your skin ask your esthetician or skin-care consultant for some guidance as well as a few complimentary samples. This will enable you to judge the compatability of the product with your skin. If you are on a budget and need to keep your spending to a minimum, the three most important products you need are a moisturizing type of cleanser, a day moisturizer, and, most important, a maximum-strength sunscreen with an SPF of 15 or higher. The reason that I did not suggest a day moisturizer that contains a sunscreen is because you will be using this product for both day and night. But if you decide to purchase a night creme (excellent in cases of extreme dry skin) then your day creme should contain a sunscreen with an SPF of 15 or higher.

TWO IMPORTANT TIPS FOR ENHANCING THE EFFECTIVENESS OF YOUR SKIN-CARE PRODUCTS

If you want to increase the permeability and absorption of your skin-care products into the stratum corneum you must follow these two points:

1. Always apply your moisturizing products (cleanser, day moisturizer, night creme, or eye creme) to your skin when it is in a fully hydrated state. Splashing or misting water on your face before you apply any moisturizing product will make it penetrate the outermost layer of your skin more efficiently than it would if your skin were dry.
2. The next important point is to exfoliate your stratum corneum; this is an effective way to enhance the effect of the skin-care products you're using. Use either an extremely fine grain scrub or a product that contains AHAs. Remember, the dead skin cell layer acts as a barrier to protect your skin. But cell turnover decreases in sun-damaged and mature skin. If you allow your complexion to accumulate too many dead skin cells, it will look dull and flaky and it will interfere with the penetration of any product into the stratum corneum.

SEEKING OUT THE PROFESSIONALS AND TREATMENTS THAT CAN HELP YOU ENHANCE YOUR COMPLEXION

Dermatologists, cosmetic surgeons, and estheticians are on the list of professions who can help guide you to a healthier, fresher-looking complexion. There are many nonmedical esthetic (skin beautifying) treatments that can help you improve the surface of your skin. There are also various medical treatments that help repair the ravaging effects of sun damage. All these freshen a maturing complexion.

Professional Facials! How They Can Make Your Complexion Look More Vibrant

If you want a professional to care for your skin in a nonmedical capacity, seek out an esthetician. These highly trained individuals practice their profession in skin-care clinics, full-service salons, day spas, destination spas, and in some dermatology and cosmetic surgeon's offices, under the supervision of a physician.

An esthetician analyzes your complexion carefully to determine your skin type and documents all the information, so your progress can be tracked. Your esthetician will ask you numerous questions about your skin and your at-home skin-care routine. Then, he or she will deliver a customized skin treatment in the form of a facial.

There are many different types of facials, and in better salons each one is uniquely tailored to suit the needs of an individual. A facial for mature or sun-damaged skin includes a deep cleansing to thoroughly remove all embedded dirt and makeup, an exfoliation in the form of either a facial scrub or an exfoliating wash of alpha hydroxy acids, a massage to relax you and temporarily improve your circulation, and a moisturizing treatment performed with a concentrated product containing high levels of emollients. All four steps have a beneficial effect on the surface (stratum corneum) of your skin; they can also boost your spirits.

Your esthetician will direct you to the correct products for your skin type and condition. In many cases, he or she may give you a sample of a skin-care product to try at home. If he or she is suggesting a costly product or product system, don't be afraid to ask for samples before you invest.

Innovative Skin Rx! Three Medical Therapies that Reduce the Effects of Aging and Sun-Damaged Skin

Dermatologists and cosmetic surgeons are highly skilled physicians who offer various medical and surgical procedures that will enhance the quality of the skin. (Medical surgical procedures and chemical peels are covered in Chapter Twelve.)

Dermatologists use three primary topical prescription ingredients to help repair sun-damaged and maturing skin to look fresher and more even in tone: retinoic acid or Retin-A, hydroquinone or bleaching cream, and prescription-strength alpha hydroxy acid. (For more detailed information about these three medical treatments refer to Chapter Twelve.)

SUN-DAMAGED SKIN—TWENTY-FOUR SERIOUS CONCERNS AND SKIN REPAIRING MEDICAL TREATMENTS

Dermatologists and cosmetic surgeons are faced with a whole host of possible life-threatening concerns and superficial problems when treating sun-damaged skin. Sun-damaged skin is the primary cause of most premature aging problems. Ultraviolet radiation affects four major areas of the skin: the pigment, elasticity, blood vessels, and texture. The entire composition of the skin is disrupted and transformed from a smooth, youthful, glowing, healthy-looking skin to a complexion that looks weathered and damaged.

The first and most serious concern that dermatologists are looking for when treating sun-damaged skin is skin cancer. Your physician will look for basal cell (most common and most treatable) and squamous cell (treatable if caught early, but it is more aggressive than basal-cell cancer). Both basal- and squamous-cell cancers have an excellent prognosis if diagnosed early. The treatment for both these types of skin cancers is either removal by a surgical procedure, cortorizing (burning) with a hot implement, or cryosurgery (freezing) with liquid nitrogen. Your doctor will also look for signs of the most deadly form of skin cancer—malignant melanoma (this aggressive form of skin cancer quickly spreads to the organs). This type of skin cancer strikes at an early age, in the thirties and forties, because it is linked to sunburns, not long-term sun exposure.

The best way to prevent skin cancer is to wear a sunscreen with an SPF of 15 or higher any time you are exposed to sunlight as well as to examine your skin regularly by following the American Academy of Dermatology examination chart on page 258.

The second factor dermatologists and cosmetic surgeons face when treating sun-damaged skin is the extensive damage to connective tissue that contributes to wrinkles, thinning of the skin, and loss of elasticity. The wrinkles can be softened with a superficial, medium, or deep chemical peel depending on the depth of the wrinkles. The loss of elasticity can be addressed and improved with cosmetic surgery (See Chapter Twelve).

Negative changes in your skin coloring can be quite dramatic depending on the accumulation of sun damage. Pigmentation problems come in various forms: freckles, liver or age spots (senile lentigines), moles, hypo-pigmentation (loss of color in areas), and hyper-pigmentation (a deepening of color in areas). Medical treatments include Retin-A, glycolic acid peels, skin lighteners (hydroquinone), chemical peels, and laser surgery (the carbon-dioxide laser-CO^2, copper vapor laser, dye lasers, and the ruby laser).

Blood vessels are affected by ultraviolet radiation. The small capillaries (tiny network of veins) that are closest to the skin are damaged by UV rays. The walls are damaged, causing a weakening of the vessels. Dilation occurs under their weakened state because the capillaries cannot withstand the pressure of the blood. A condition call telangrectasia develops that causes a spidery-looking network of small red veins. If sun exposure is extensive a chronic reddening (erythema) could take place. The capillaries become permanently dilated so that the skin takes on a red and blotchy look in these areas. The most popular medical treatments for these vascular sun-related conditions are laser treatments (including argon laser, copper laser, and dye laser).

"AGE-BUSTING" TIPS THAT WILL HELP KEEP YOUR SKIN YOUNG

Preserving a more youthful complexion is easier and less expensive than you think. Preventative care can help you avoid the skin abuse that causes premature aging or can aggravate the skin. Here are a few simple, cost effective, age-busting tips that you can use every day at home to help you preserve a youthful complexion.

Protect Your Skin from the Sun

Aging and gravity are tough enough on your precious, protective covering—your skin. Why compound the problem with the most severe environmental trauma of sun exposure? Unprotected sun exposure can add 10 to 15 years to your skin's appearance, and all the moisturizers, night treatments, and eye cremes in the world won't cover up the damage. Everyone talks about special treatments for sun-damaged skin, but my most valuable advice involves prevention.

Sun-damage prevention comes in many forms, including avoiding the sun, correctly applying a sunscreen with an SPF of 15 or higher, and wearing tightly woven, protective clothing, wide-brimmed hats, and UV-tested sunglasses. True, there are several treatments for sun-damaged skin that are effective, but it is futile to spend time and money to treat sun damage if you continue to cause it.

Avoid Tugging or Pulling When You Are Cleansing or Moisturizing Your Face

Your method of cleansing your face should be as gentle as it would be if you were washing a delicate peach. When you reach the age of 30, your skin becomes more delicate and injury prone.

Preserving your skin's natural tone and elasticity should be one of your first skin-care priorities. Tugging or pulling your face, eyes, or throat adds wear and tear to your skin. Keep this in mind the next time you cleanse, exfoliate, or apply moisturizer. You are not scrubbing a kitchen floor, sanding your outdoor furniture, or applying furniture polish to your dining room table. Your skin is a living organ, not an inanimate object, so be gentle.

Treat your skin gently with the following routine:

A. Splash your face with warm water before you apply your cleanser. The cleanser will spread more easily on premoistened skin, eliminating the need for pulling or tugging.

B. If your skin is sensitive, use a smooth sponge to cleanse your face instead of a terry washcloth. The smooth surface of the sponge will gently glide over your delicate skin without causing much friction.

C. Take extra care when you remove your eye makeup or apply eye-care products because the skin around the eyes is extremely thin. The rule I like to follow is to always work your way inward, toward the nose, when cleansing the eye area or applying moisturizer.

D. When removing your makeup, use a 100 percent cotton eye pad. Moisten it with water, then split it in half and dispense a small amount of cleanser or fragrance-free eye makeup remover onto the eye pad. Next, gently apply the cotton to the eye area, hold it in place for a moment, then sweep it over the skin. Use very little pressure. Repeat this action until the eye area is free of makeup.

Tugging, rubbing, and pulling don't expedite the removal of makeup; in fact, moving hastily and quickly is counterproductive because it takes time for the product to break down mascara and eye makeup. Think of removing your eye makeup as using a semi-compress technique. Holding the eye pad on the skin for just a moment maximizes the effectiveness of the cleanser or eye-makeup remover.

Apply Eye Creams with Extra Care

Grinding moisturizer into the skin doesn't make it work more effectively; it deters the action of the product. Use your pinkie or ring finger in a gentle patting motion when you apply product to the eye area. This technique is safe for delicate skin because those two fingers don't have the same strength your index finger does.

Quench Your Skin's Thirst for Moisture

The production of your skin's natural oils slows as you age. This change interferes with your skin's ability to hold moisture. Without moisture, your skin becomes dehydrated and shows symptoms of tightness and flakiness.

Moisturizers help to plump up the stratum corneum with water and emollients, which can transform dry, parched, tight-looking skin into a complexion that appears fresher. The beneficial effects will last for only a few hours; their longevity also depends on your environment. If your indoor air is dry and hot, or if it is extremely cold outdoors, the drying process will be expedited.

Moisturize your skin on a daily basis and you'll help your skin preserve its natural moisture. If you use a moisturizer with an SPF of 15 or higher, you're giving your skin double the protection. This simple step takes only a minute, so no matter how busy you are, it's easy to make moisturizing part of your daily routine. When you do, follow these moisturizing tips:

A. Maximize the effectiveness of your moisturizer by applying it to premoistened skin. Splash your face with water or with an alcohol-free toner. This facilitates a frictionless, even distribution of the moisturizing product.
B. Don't forget to moisturize your throat and your décolleté. I count these areas as part of the facial area because they are so visible and exposed. An unpampered throat and décolleté can cause you to look older than your true age, so the next time you moisturize your face, dispense a little extra product and moisturize these areas too. Always use upward strokes and work in the opposite direction of gravity.
C. Enhance the moisturizing process by using a product that contains alpha hydroxy acids.

Exfoliate the Dull Skin Away

As you age, your skin's cellular turnover slows down. This, in turn, interferes with the natural shedding ability of the stratum corneum, causing your skin to appear dull, pasty, and flaky. Facial scrubs or over-the-counter alpha hydroxy acids products that remove dead skin cells can improve the superficial texture of your skin when used over a period of time.

Avoid Hot Showers and Baths

Using extremely hot water when bathing can irritate your skin and rob it of natural oils. Use only tepid-to-warm water and hold showers to 10 minutes or less if you are experiencing dry, itchy, flaky skin. When you are in the shower, apply a body oil to your moistened skin and avoid deodorant soaps. They can irritate dry skin. If you are taking a bath, add a few capfuls of bath oil to your bath water. This will help to keep your skin soft.

Add Moisture to Your Environment

Humidifiers can help replenish moisture in the air of your home, making it a more friendly atmosphere for your skin. If the air around you is dry, it will rob moisture from your skin through evaporation.

Smooth "Alligator" Skin

Occasionally, the skin on your body can become extremely dry, scaly, or even itchy. Applying moisturizer doesn't always correct the problem. You may need to use an abrasive loofah sponge or an exfoliating mitt or glove. This will help polish and slough off dead, flaky skin cells on your body. While you shower, apply a body oil to wet skin, then moisten the loofah, glove, or mitt and massage your skin, starting with your feet, working upward and ending with your décolleté. Rinse well, then apply a rich body creme or oil while your skin is still moist.

Get Quality Sleep to Refresh and Rejuvenate Your Skin

If lack of sleep makes you feel irritable, imagine what it does to your skin. Sleepless nights can trigger the kind of stress that causes your skin to look dull, puffy, tired, or sallow. The skin around your eyes may look a little more crepy in texture. Sleep can be your best beauty remedy. Each night, sleep gives your skin a mini-vacation and time to renew itself.

Avoid Dry Lips Which Can Reveal Your True Age

There is nothing more frustrating than having your lipstick feather around your lip line. This is a problem that occurs when your skin is on the dry side. The skin around your lips draws moisture from the lipstick, and the color of the product is drawn into the fine lines around the natural lip line. This accentuates any fine lines or wrinkles you may have. Try this:

- Exfoliate your lips when you exfoliate your face.
- Apply an extra application of moisturizer on your lips before you apply your foundation and lip color.
- Apply a light application of foundation over your lips to act as a primer for the lip color.
- Line your lips with a lip pencil and finish with a softer shade of lip color. (The waxy consistency of the lip pencil will help to control and block the feathering of the lip color past your natural lip line. Lighter shades of lip color downplay this problem area more than darker shades do.)

Avoid Aging Hands

Often, hands give away your age, particularly if they show age spots, rough skin, or brittle nails. Prematurely aging hands don't mix with a youthful face. Your hands are exposed to daily abuse, but there are simple and inexpensive precautions you can take to preserve your hands' youthful appearance:

- When you apply your sunscreen with an SPF of 15 or higher (on a daily basis), don't forget to apply it all over your hands. Your hands are one of the most exposed areas of your body, and they are highly prone to sun damage. The daily use of sunscreen will slow the development of age spots on your hands and arms.
- Exfoliate your hands with your facial scrub to help slough away rough dry skin.
- Maintain smooth skin by using a hand creme that contains alpha hydroxy acids.
- Have a weekly manicure.
- Brittle-looking nails with ridges can be gently buffed, creating a smoother, healthier finish. Use a nonacetone polish remover

and a nail polish that contain no formaldehyde to prevent nails from drying out.

- Follow the no-nonsense skin-care program that fits any busy lifestyle (see Chapter Three).

LEARN HOW TO CHANGE YOUR SKIN-CARE HABITS

Once your skin begins to mature, you cannot follow the same skin-care routine or use the same products you did you when you were in your late teens or twenties. Your skin has different needs now, and slight adjustments may be necessary. Here are a few simple changes that can have a positive effect on your skin:

- If your skin is on the dry side, use an alcohol-free toner instead of an astringent.
- Switch to a cleansing lotion or cream instead of an oil-free gel, which is designed for normal to oily skin.
- Never use harsh or abrasive facial scrubs. Use mild, gentle facial scrubs with microscopic grains, or use a product that contains alpha hydroxy acids.
- Never skip the moisturizing step of skin care. If your skin still feels dry after moisturizing, you may need to switch to a richer type of cream moisturizer.
- Pay special attention to the most delicate zone on your face, the eye area. Wear sunglasses outside year-round to avoid squinting. A special eye creme may be necessary as a dry-skin remedy for around your eyes. Apply this product every morning and night.
- Follow a complete skin-care routine twice a day by cleansing, toning, and moisturizing and by using an eye creme and a lip balm with a high SPF factor.
- Once or twice a week give yourself a complete facial, including use of an exfoliant and a masque (see Chapter Three) that are designed for your particular skin type (see Chapter Two). It

may take a few extra minutes, but you are helping your skin reach its true potential.

- If your skin is excessively dry, night creme may be a necessary addition to your skin-care regimen. Night cremes are richer in consistency than day moisturizers and can soften your skin while you sleep. When you awaken, your skin will feel replenished instead of parched.
- If you suffer from excessively dry skin, it may be necessary to cleanse your skin only at night to remove your makeup. In the morning, use an alcohol-free toner before applying your moisturizer.

SUM IT UP!

As you can see after reading this chapter, seeking the "fountain of youth" is not found in some exotic, mysterious place halfway around the world or in some expensive skin-care jar. Actually, it is quite inexpensive and easier than you think. What is the secret component that holds the key to prolonging your youthful complexion? **PREVENTION!** And you are the only one in control. Prevention is the best anti-aging prescription you have to help ward off Father Time. There are a great many excellent medical skin rejuvenation procedures and prescriptions as well as plenty of over-the-counter skin-care products for mature and sun-damaged skin, but it is difficult to treat sun damage if you are still causing trauma to your skin with unprotected sun exposure.

Aging is inevitable, so why add insult to injury by accelerating the natural process of life prematurely? If you act as a responsible "caretaker" of your skin by examining your skin regularly and shielding yourself and loved ones with a sunscreen (SPF 15 or higher) from a true environmental hazard—the sun—you can prevent a great deal (up to 80 percent to 90 percent if you were shielded as a child) of premature aging that is caused by sun damage. Just think, you could be wearing the effects of your sun exposure today as fine lines, wrinkles, and sagging skin tomorrow, or even worse, you could be faced with skin cancer. It is up to you!

CHAPTER *Ten*

TANNING
THE GOOD AND THE BAD

It's time to come to grips with the fact that the days of roasting or even walking in the sun without proper skin protection are over. But do you still love that "healthy" tanned look even though you're aware that the sun causes premature aging? If you answer yes, it is time to discuss the safe way to create a deep, dark tropical tan without being anywhere near the sun. This chapter will introduce you to the dynamics of protecting yourself and your family from the harmful rays of the sun. It will teach you how to select an appropriate sun-protection product (sunscreens) for your skin tone and how the SPF factor actually protects the skin. You will explore the options of "sunless tanning" with innovative self-tanning products. And you will receive information and recommendations about the sun from the American Academy of Dermatology.

HISTORICALLY SPEAKING—DISCOVER WHY OUR ANCESTORS GRAVITATED TO THE SUN

Human fascination with the sun began thousands of years ago when our ancestors worshipped the sun as a god. It was the center of their universe and their only source of energy. They depended on it for light, warmth, and comfort.

This love for the sun came into the twentieth century in the form of a beauty ritual. People thought they looked healthy if they had a tan. They flocked to the beach to roast, baste, and broil. They drenched their skin in suntan oils so they could fry until well done. (Remember baby oil with iodine?) The goal was to achieve that perfect tan during a one- or two-week vacation. Peeling skin (like a snake shedding its skin) became a summer ritual. It was thought that lobsterlike skin was the pain to be endured to get the ultimate golden glow.

How did this phenomenon begin? In the fifties, tanned skin was in. Magazines promoted the sexy look of a tan—you know, the "California tan." If you were pale during the summer months you felt like an outcast. But little did anyone know that an invisible trauma was taking place. That's right! A tan is trauma and injury to the skin.

Today, we still gravitate to the sun. A sunny day puts us in a good mood; the warmth of the sun is comforting and relaxing. A beautiful sunrise and sunset is breathtaking and even romantic. Many of our recreational activities are focused around a sunny day. The growth of our food supply and plant life on earth depends on the sun. How can something so important to our well-being be so harmful to our health?

TEST YOUR SUN KNOWLEDGE IQ

In addition to being life-giving and romantic, the sun can be ruthless. The sun can bake and crack the earth in the summer. It can fade the color of our curtains, carpets, and paint. It can peel the paint on our houses, melt or crack the tar in our streets, evaporate the water in our reservoirs, and ignite a spark through a prism or glass. If the sun can erode our terrain and dwellings in this way, just think what it can do to our skin.

How much do you know about protecting your skin from sun damage? Take this test and find out!

Sun Test

1. As long as I don't get a sunburn I don't have to worry about the sun.

   True False

2. Applying sunscreen before going outdoors will protect me all day.

   True False

3. Cloudy days protect us from the sun, so no sunscreen is needed.

   True False

4. Mediterranean or darker skin types do not need sun protection because they don't burn.

   True False

5. Avoiding the sun for a few years will guarantee that no wrinkles or skin cancer will develop.

   True False

6. Tanning parlors and sun lamps are a safe alternative for tanning. If there is no sun there will be no skin damage.

   True False

7. If I get a tan from a self-tan product, I don't need to use sunscreen.

   True False

Answers: All sun sleuths know that all these statements are False! How'd you do? Now keep reading to find out the why and how of each of these points.

STOP THE AGING—RUN FOR COVER

Because sun damage is invisible to the naked eye, there are still many people who don't take unprotected sun exposure seriously, despite constant media warnings about the sun. You know the expression "Out of sight out of mind." What do you think would happen if we could actually see the UV rays of the sun penetrating our skin like little bullets or lasers? You can bet we would all run for cover. Clothing manufacturers would be scurrying around to design protective yet fashionable suits of armor.

Sound dramatic? Not really; far too many people suffer from the "It can't happen to me syndrome." This is a serious affliction that caused 700,000 new cases of skin cancer in the United States in

1994 according to the American Academy of Dermatology. One in six Americans will develop skin cancer in his or her lifetime.

I'm going to give unprotected sun exposure a new label. Let's call it "Skin Abuse" because it is overindulgence of a substance (the sun) that is known to harm your health. And if you think you're safe because you don't get a sunburn and you only allow yourself to tan gradually, you're sadly mistaken—there is no such thing as a "little trauma" to the skin. Only time will tell just how much damage was caused by your sun exposure.

FOUR SURPRISING FACTS ABOUT YOUR SKIN AND THE SUN

Many people have a false sense of security about their vulnerability to sun damage. Do any of these statements sound familiar?

1. "I get tan only on my one vacation a year."
2. "I haven't gotten a tan or lain out in the sun since I was a teenager or young adult."
3. "I received only one or two bad sunburns in my entire life."
4. "I allow myself to develop a tan only gradually; I never sunburn."

All these people have received enough UVA and UVB exposure to cause sun damage. All you need is one bad sunburn to start you on your way to premature aging and even worse—skin cancer. And, if your skin tans buts never burns you have still caused skin damage. If you have been avoiding the sun in recent years, you're not out of the woods because most skin damage occurs from sun exposure we received as a child.

SEVEN TIPS TO HELP YOU PREVENT SKIN CANCER

The American Academy of Dermatology recommends the following precautions to lessen the chances of developing skin cancer:

1. **Minimize sun exposure,** especially during the peak sun hours of 10 A.M. to 4 P.M., when solar radiation is most intense.
2. **Wear appropriate clothing** during prolonged periods in the sun—tight textile weave, long sleeves, pants, and a full-brim hat.
3. **Protect children** by keeping them out of the sun, especially those under six months old. Minimize sun exposure whenever possible and apply sunscreens to children older than six months.
4. **Apply sunscreen or sunblock liberally and frequently,** and reapply every two hours when working, playing, or exercising outdoors. A product with a sun protection factor (SPF) of at least 15 is recommended, even on overcast days when 80 percent of the sun's rays may penetrate the clouds.
5. **Beware of reflective surfaces.** Sand, snow, concrete, and water can reflect up to 85 percent of the sun's damaging rays.
6. **Avoid tanning salons and sun lamps.** The ultraviolet radiation emitted by these artificial sources is similar to that of sunlight and can cause sunburn, premature skin aging, and an increased risk of skin cancers.
7. **Teach children and teens about sun protection** because skin damage from sun exposure accumulates over a lifetime. (Most of a person's lifetime sun damage occurs before age 20.) One or more blistering childhood or adolescent sunburns can double the risk of developing malignant melanoma, a lethal form of skin cancer.

Detect skin cancer at its earliest, most curable stage. Examine your skin regularly, and other family members too, for any changes to freckles or moles or new skin discolorations. Learn the early warning signs of skin cancer. See the Periodic Self-Examination instructions on page 258. If any disturbing change is noticed, or a strange new spot appears, see your dermatologist immediately.

Tanning and Skin Trauma Are One and the Same

There is no safe way to tan with UV rays. A suntan is the skin's response to an injury. Tanning occurs when the sun's ultraviolet

Periodic Self-Examination

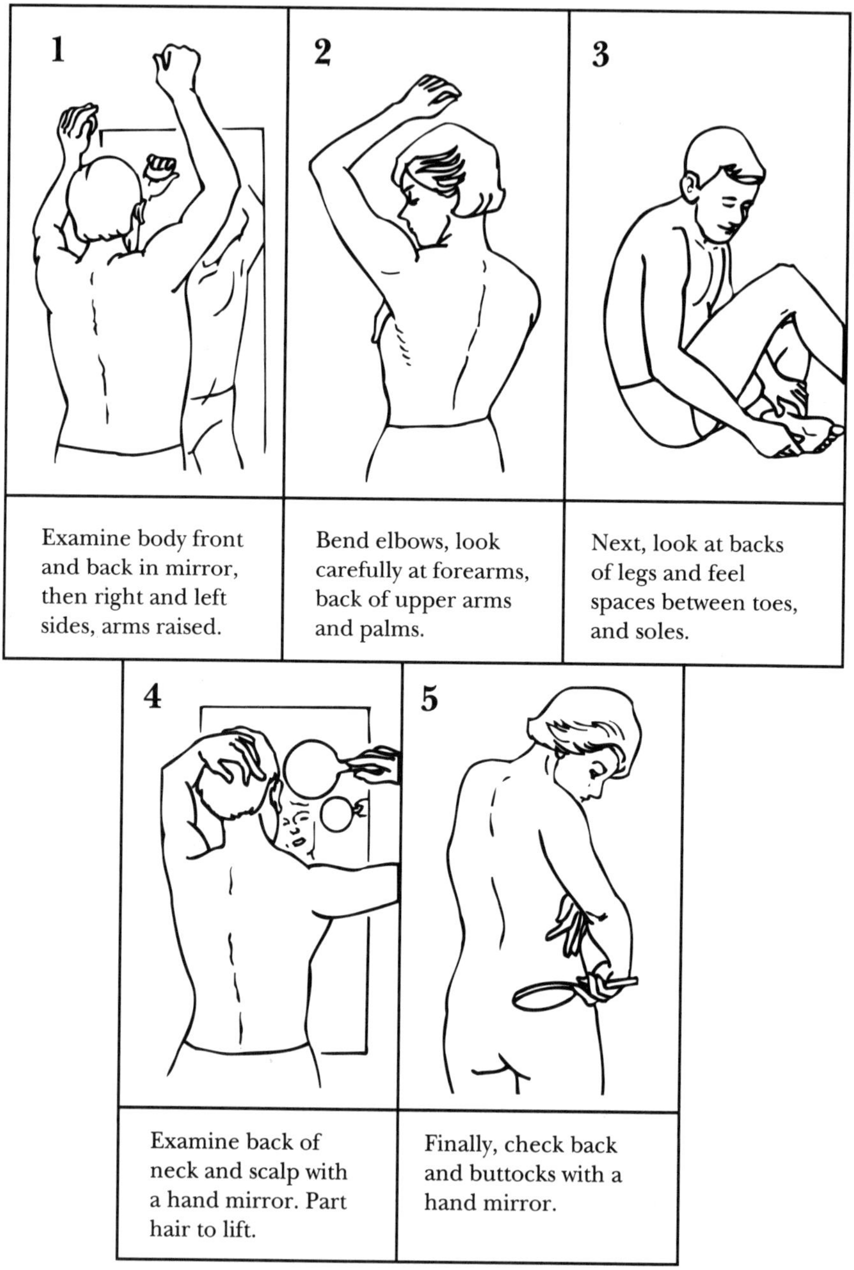

Figure 9 Courtesy of The American Academy of Dermatology.

rays penetrate the skin's inner layer, which causes the skin to produce more melanin (the pigment that gives the skin its color) as a response to the injury. It also affects the connective tissue (which gives the skin its shape) by making it less toned. Chronic exposure to the sun can cause sun damage (see Chapter Nine, Timeless Beauty), which results in a change in the skin's texture, tone, and blood vessels, causing wrinkling, age spots, and a leathered look as well as loose, sagging skin, red blotches, and dilated capillaries.

Tanning Booths—Watch Out!

In spite of claims that tanning booths offer "safe" tanning havens, exposure in these booths can cause cataracts (eye damage), sunburns, skin cancer, and premature aging of the skin. Tanning booths emit UVA radiation, which can pose both short- and long-term risks to the skin. Artificial radiation carries all the risks of real sunlight.

Damage to the Immune System

Your body's natural line of defense, your immune system, can be affected by the UVA rays emitted by tanning lights. Ultraviolet light has a negative effect on the immune system because many of the immune cells are located in the skin, which makes them an easy target. The UVA rays that cause a burn or tan will not only harm your skin but they will also harm the immune cells that protect you from viruses and bacteria. When the immune system is damaged, you become more susceptible to infection and diseases.

Beware Photsensitizing Substances There are quite a few over-the-counter medications, prescription drugs (oral contraceptives, tetracyclines, sulfonamides, diuretics, and tranquilizers, to name a few), artificial sweeteners, food preservatives, cosmetics, detergents, and essential oils from plants and flowers (as used in perfumes) that can exacerbate ultraviolet damage. These internal and external products are called photosensitizing substances. They trigger a response in the skin cells that sends a message to absorb an increased amount of UV rays from either tanning booths or the sun. The result is an intensified reaction to the ultraviolet light that induces either an inflammation or an oozing and crusting of the skin. If you are taking prescription drugs always read the labels on the bottle because the pharmacist will post a warning alerting you to possible photosensitive reaction. If you are being treated with a photosensitizing drug, it is extremely important to avoid tanning parlors.

Unregulated Parlors

Many tanning parlors are unregulated, allowing customers access to tanning beds without supervision or eye protection. (This is especially dangerous for those with sun-sensitive skin.) The American Academy of Dermatology has launched a campaign for the introduction of local and/or statewide tanning-parlor legislation. Among other possible regulatory provisions, this legislation would require that warning signs be prominently displayed in tanning parlors with a list of the hazards of such exposure.

KEEP YOUR SKIN YOUNG—DISCOVER THE BEST ANTI-AGING PRODUCTS YOU CAN BUY

The best anti-aging products are sunscreens. In fact, there are many cosmetic products available today that contain sunscreens for daily use because sun protection is the principal means of preventing premature aging and skin cancer. Sunscreens used on a regular basis actually allow some repair of damage skin.

YOU CAN HAVE FLAWLESS SKIN—FACTS ABOUT SUNSCREENS YOU SHOULD KNOW

(Courtesy of The American Academy of Dermatology)

The SPF Factor

SPF stands for *Sun Protection Factor.* Sunscreens are rated or classified in this manner. They have SPF numbers on their packaging that range from 2 to as high as 50. These numbers refer to the product's ability to screen or block out the sun's burning rays.

SPFs are determined by scientific testing in a laboratory. Using a machine that simulates sunlight, a small patch of a volunteer's skin is exposed to sunburn rays without a sunscreen to determine how much sunlight will cause a mild sunburn. Similar exposure is done on an area of the skin covered with sunscreen. Then scientists compare the amount of time needed to produce a sunburn on protected skin to the amount of time needed to cause a sunburn on the unprotected skin. For example, if a sunscreen is rated SPF 2 and a fair-skinned person who would normally turn red after 10 minutes of exposure in the sun uses it, it would take 20 minutes of exposure for the skin to turn red. A sunscreen with an SPF of 15 would allow that person to multiply that initial burning time by 15 minutes, which means it would take 15 times longer to burn, or 150 minutes. Dermatologists strongly recommend a sunscreen with an SPF of 15 or greater year-round for all skin types.

Consumers be aware that SPF protection does not increase proportionally with a designated SPF number. In higher SPFs, such as an SPF of 34, 97 percent of sun-burning rays are absorbed, while an SPF of 15 indicates 93 percent absorption, and an SPF of 2 allows 50 percent absorption.

The Dark-Skin Myth

The FDA (Food and Drug Administration) and the American Academy of Dermatology recognize six skin categories based on the rate at which the skin burns. Skin types 4, 5, and 6 minimally or rarely burn and so often are left unprotected. But regardless of skin type, the American Academy of Dermatology suggests that *all* people use a sunscreen year-round with an SPF of at least 15.

PABA News

PABA, or para-aminobenzoic acid, was the original compound that was the basic ingredient in sunscreens. However, it stains clothes. Today, PABA has been refined and the newer ingredients called PABA esters include glycerol PABA, padimate A (pentyl dimethyl

PABA), and padimate O (octyl dimethyl PABA). These rarely stain clothing as PABA once did. Some people are sensitive to PABA and other ingredients commonly found in sunscreens such as benzophenones (oxybenzone), cinnamates (octylmethyl cinnamate and cinoxate), and salicylates.

UVA and UVB Light Wavelengths and How They Affect Your Skin

Sunlight consists of two types of harmful rays: UVB rays and UVA rays. The UVB rays are the sun's burning rays (which are blocked by window glass) and are the primary cause of sunburn and skin cancer. UVA rays (which pass through window glass) penetrate déeper into the dermis (second layer of the skin), or base layer of the skin. UVA rays in addition to UVB rays are the culprits in premature wrinkling of the skin and also contribute toward skin burning and skin cancer.

Since PABA, PABA esters, and cinnamates protect against only UVB light, check a sunscreen for ingredients that also screen UVA rays, such as benzophenones, oxybenzone, sulisobenzone, titanium dioxide, zinc oxide, and Parsol 1789 (butyl methoxydibenzoylmethane, also called avobenzone). These are also known as broad-spectrum sunscreens.

Note: The SPF number on a sunscreen reflects the product's screening ability only for UVB rays. At the present time there is no FDA-approved rating system that identifies UVA protection.

Using a cream, oil, or lotion is a matter of personal choice, but keep in mind that most oils do not contain sufficient amounts of sunscreens and usually have an SPF of less than 2. All sunscreens need to be reapplied. Gels sweat off and wash off more easily and therefore need to be applied more frequently, but they may be preferable for acne-prone people.

Daily Use

Sunscreens can be used every day if you are going to be in the sun for more than 20 minutes, and that also includes driving in your car. They can be applied under makeup. There are many cosmetic products available today that contain sunscreens for daily use because sun protection is the principal means of preventing premature aging and skin cancer. Sunscreens used on a regular basis actually allow some repair of damaged skin.

Because the sun's reflective powers are great (17 percent on sand and 80 percent on snow), don't reserve the use of these products for sunny summer days. Even on a cloudy day, 80 percent of the sun's ultraviolet rays pass through the clouds.

EIGHT EFFECTIVE SUNSCREEN-APPLICATION TECHNIQUES

1. Sunscreens should be applied to dry skin 15 to 30 minutes *before* going outdoors.
2. Apply your sunscreen liberally (one ounce is considered enough to cover the entire body) and pay particular attention to the face, hands, and arms.
3. Be careful to cover exposed areas completely. A missed spot could mean a patchy, painful sunburn.
4. Lips get sunburned too, so apply a lip product that contains sunscreen with an SPF of 15.
5. Sunscreens should be applied in the morning and reapplied after swimming or perspiring heavily.
6. Even so-called waterproof sunscreens may lose their effectiveness after 80 minutes in the water.
7. Sunscreens rub off as well as wash off, so if you've towel-dried or have been in the water for longer than 80 minutes, reapply your waterproof sunscreen for maximum protection.
8. Remember that sun exposure occurs all the time, even during a lunchtime stroll on a cloudy afternoon.

SIX NO-FAIL WAYS TO RESCUE YOUR SUNBURNED SKIN

In case you forgot to cover up and apply your sunscreen and find yourself with a sunburn, remember that it *can* be dangerous. There are two types of sunburns you should know about.

First-Degree Sunburn

- Will cause redness and some peeling and will heal within a few days.
- First-degree burns can be painful and are best treated with cool baths and bland moisturizer (unscented) or over-the-counter hydrocortisone creams.
- Aspirin taken orally may lessen early development of a sunburn.

Second-Degree Burn

- This type of blistering burn can be considered a medical emergency if a large area of your body is affected.
- When a burn is severe, accompanied by a headache, chills, or fever, seek medical help immediately.
- Be sure to protect your skin from the sun while it heals and thereafter.

SEVEN SURPRISING FACTS ON OZONE AND HOW IT RELATES TO SKIN CANCER

1. Does the depletion of stratospheric ozone by manmade chlorofluorocarbons (CFCs) have any effect on skin cancer incidence?

   Not at the present because there is a 10- to 20-year time lag between exposure to ultraviolet light and the development of skin malignancy. But scientists do expect some increase in skin cancer in the future due to ozone depletion caused by CFCs.

2. What are CFCs, and why can't all countries ban them?

   Chlorofluorocarbons (CFCs) were developed in 1930 as safe alternatives to toxic and flammable refrigerants that were being used at the time. CFCs are chemically unique compounds that are nonreactive and have very useful chemical properties. They are nontoxic to humans and yet have ideal vaporization temperatures for air conditioning and for expanding plastic foam used as insulation for appliances and buildings. They are also excellent cleaning agents for delicate electronic and mechanical instruments. CFCs are relatively simple and inexpensive to manufacture, while substitutes are much more expensive to produce and therefore more costly for developing countries.

3. How does ozone affect the amount of ultraviolet radiation that reaches the earth?

   The ozone filter is a crucial protection against the carcinogenic impact of sunlight on humans. Ozone blocks ultraviolet C from reaching the earth's surface and blocks significant amounts of ultraviolet B radiation that damages DNA, but has little effect on ultraviolet A radiation. Recent data have shown that there is a recurrent ozone hole in the stratosphere over Antarctica in which ozone levels have been reduced as much as 60 percent some years. Atmospheric concentrations of trace gases such as carbon dioxide, methane, nitrous oxide, and CFCs have been increasing at an alarming rate.

4. Will ozone depletion produce more skin cancer?

   Yes. A 1988 U.S. EPA (Environmental Protection Agency) study estimated that a 1 percent decrease in atmospheric ozone could cause a 4 to 6 percent increase in nonmelanoma skin cancers in Americans born before 2070.

5. How does this translate in terms of new cases of skin cancers?

   Unless there are controls on the causes of ozone depletion, estimates are that there could possibly be 163 to 310 million additional nonmelanoma skin cancers and 840,000 to 1.4 million additional melanomas, which could result in an estimated 3.2 million deaths by 2075. Even modest reductions of ozone could result in an increased incidence of nonmelanoma and melanoma skin cancers.

6. Have these changes taken place yet?

   There has not yet been a significant measurable change in ultraviolet B radiation as a consequence of CFCs in the stratosphere in the United States. However, this may be related to air pollution and aerosols in the atmosphere screening out the ultraviolet rays.

7. What other changes would there be if no controls were imposed?

   Increased radiation from the sun could affect phytoplankton in the ocean. These small plants are responsible for 66 percent of the photosynthesis occurring on earth by which carbon dioxide is exchanged for oxygen. This could enhance the "greenhouse effect" and possibly reduce the quality of the air humans breathe. Animal plankton, the food staple for many forms of ocean animal life, is also vulnerable to increased levels of ultraviolet B radiation. Ultraviolet B radiation is known to decrease the growth of most known plant species, and further ozone depletion could result in a decrease in the variety of plant life. However, exactly what would happen to the food chain is not clear at this time.

THE AMERICAN ACADEMY OF DERMATOLOGY SPEAKS OUT ABOUT SUN PROTECTION

SPF for Kids Not High Enough, AAD Says
Dermatologists critique FDA's sunscreen monograph

Schaumburg, IL—May 2, 1994—In comments recently submitted to the Food and Drug Administration (FDA) on behalf of the Academy, AAD President Peyton E. Weary, M.D., disputed the agency's proposed category designations for sunscreen products and suggested other changes to the monograph as well.

The Academy took issue with the FDA's minimum recommendations of a sun protection factor (SPF 4 for young children between six months and two years of age). Dr. Weary pointed out that the risk of skin reactions to sunscreen product ingredients in children is very small compared to the potential for early sun damage. Dermatologists have consistently emphasized that the bulk of most people's sun exposure occurs during their youth—usually before age 20. And a number of studies have linked skin cancers later in life to severe early sunburns.

AAD experts in the area of skin and ultraviolet exposure—photobiology—feel strongly that young children should have the benefit of the same maximum sunscreen protection as others. Says Dr. John Epstein, a member of the AAD's Environmental Council,

"If children older than six months are going to be out of doors any significant amount of time, they should be encouraged to use more potent sunscreens." (The AAD advises that the skin of infants younger than six months is best shielded with appropriated clothing and/or sun avoidance.)

The AAD's public education efforts continue to target children with sun protection messages. An award-winning Joel Mole teaches children through posters and public service announcements to cover up, seek shade, or use sun protection when their shadows are shorter than they are.

In the monograph's recommendations for older children and adults, the AAD believes the FDA doesn't go far enough. FDA proposes to characterize sunscreen SPFs in the manner below, but dermatologists have agreed for years that the minimum acceptable sunscreen is an SPF 15. ADD membership is concerned that classifying SPF 15 as "high" would be sending the American public the wrong message, especially in view of studies that show people often do not apply enough sunscreen to do the job, or reapply as often as necessary based on their outdoor activity.

Coverage	**FDA Ranges**	**AAD — Recommended Ranges**
Minimal	SPF 2–4	SPF 4–8
Moderate	SPF 4–8	SPF 8–12
Good	—	SPF 15
High	SPF 8–12	SPF 16–30
Very High	SPF 12–20	above
Ultra	SPF 20–30	—

Other issues discussed in AAD's response to the monograph include stressing the distinction between sunscreens and sunblocks and the need for a "sun alert" label on the class of products known as sunless tanners.

Sunscreens contain special ingredients that absorb ultraviolet radiation and render it harmless. Sunscreen potency can be demonstrated and measured in laboratory testing. SPFs are an industry-wide, standardized quantification of how long specific skin types can remain in the sun without burning. Sunblocks are products containing ingredients like titanium dioxide, which physically block UV radiation. However, the amount of sun protection these provide, while potentially high, cannot be quantified in the same manner as sunscreen SPFs.

Sunless tanning products that provide a more cosmetically acceptable skin color have become popular in recent years. Most of these products contain the ingredient DHA (dihydroxyacetone). A few products provide both artificial color and some UV protection, but a "sun alert" label would warn consumers that these tanning products contain no sunscreens or sunblocks and will not keep their skin from burning.

While sunscreens and blocks are an important part of an outdoor protection regimen, dermatologists continue to stress that sun avoidance, tighter-weave clothing, long sleeves and hats with wide brims are equally necessary to avoid long-term harmful effects of UV radiation.

SURPRISE—YOUR CLOTHING CAN BE AN IMPORTANT SECOND LINE OF DEFENSE AGAINST THE SUN

Courtesy of The American Academy of Dermatology

Certain Types of Clothes Offer Better Sun Protection

New York, NY—November 15, 1994—A small but growing body of research exists that evaluates the effectiveness of various types of clothing against the harmful ultraviolet radiation (UVR) present in sunlight. Darrell Rigel, M.D., Clinical Assistant Professor of Dermatology at New York University Medical School, offered some guidelines as to what types of clothing might be preferable when a person needs to spend a lot of time outdoors. Dr. Rigel spoke to members of the news media at Dermatology Update, an Academy-sponsored seminar in New York.

Dr. Rigel explained that since the inception of its effort to educate the public about the dangers of too much UV light, the AAD has emphasized three essential components of good sun protection.

- Avoiding the sun whenever possible, especially between peak hours of 10 A.M. and 4 P.M.
- Wearing protective clothing, with long sleeves and hats and sunglasses whenever practical.

- Use of sunscreens or blockers with a sun protection factor (SPF) of 15 or greater on all exposed skin areas.

Good sun protection doesn't have to be costly, Dr. Rigel said. "Many people already have the right kind of clothing in their closets. Both natural and man-made fibers can be very effective, whether they're cotton, wool and silk, or acrylic and polyester."

Dr. Rigel added, "If you're not sure, hold the fabric up to a window or lamp and see how much light is shining through. Wearing mesh fabric or weaves with large gaps may not protect you from sunburn. And studies show the amount of protection depends on whether it's wet or dry. Which means that putting the wet T-shirt on your kids when they're at the beach may not do the trick.

Spectrophotometric and skin testing performed on various fabrics at the sun damage-causing wavelengths shows that fabrics like polyester crepe are so inadequate that normal skin will sunburn through them. On the other hand, tightly-woven cotton twills or silks, and luster polyesters can be very protective. Confusing the issue also is that relative thickness and thinness of fabric may not be relevant. A smooth-textured, satiny silk that's thin but shiny may actually reflect radiation off the fabric. The more irregular a weave, the lower the SPF on many fabrics.

Dacron polyesters may offer the most protection among man-made fabrics, while rayon, a viscose fiber, might be adequate for some people but risky for those with special skin disorders that make them more sensitive to light, such as lupus erythematosus, porphyria, or polymorphic light eruption (PLE). People with these disorders can consult their physicians about obtaining clothing items (generally available by mail order) that are tested for increased sun protection and sometimes specially treated with resins with fluorescent brighteners that absorb UV, or that have added titanium dioxide to the fabric, which keeps light from penetrating.

Dr. Rigel stated that there is a "happy medium" to seek on this issue. While most Americans aren't covering up enough when out in the sun, there is a small risk among the elderly that they will cover up too much, since this group also has the greatest number of skin cancers. "Some senior citizens who hardly ever go outdoors might not get enough sunlight on their skin for the body to produce adequate amounts of vitamin D. But this would be unusal . . . most of us get plenty of sunshine."

Hats are a fashion statement the dermatologists encourage, preferably those with a two- or three-inch brim. A study of different hat styles used by farmers found no ideal solution to the baseball cap problem: Mesh-weave caps can allow burns on balding scalps, and don't protect ears. One practical solution for outdoor workers is a style with a larger front brim and a removable back flap that covers the ears and neck. Unfortunately many hats cannot protect the lower face.

STAY YOUNG LOOKING—DISCOVER THE SAFE TWENTY-FIRST CENTURY "SUNLESS" TAN

Does a safe sunless tan sound too good to be true? Well, it's not. You can achieve a sunless glow by using self-tanning products. Please don't turn a deaf ear because you or your friends tried a similar product years ago that turned your skin orange. I promise you that the self-tanning products of today are greatly improved; they are as close as you can get to a natural-looking tan if you follow all the directions. It is worth giving this type of product a chance, especially if it is going to keep you out of the sun. Self-tan products are the only truly safe way to tan.

The Mystery Ingredient in Self-Tan Products

The active ingredient that has improved the function of today's self-tanning products is called dihydroxyacetone (DHA). It has been defined in the cosmetic industry as a colorless dye and has been approved as safe by the FDA (Food and Drug Administration). When a self-tan product containing this ingredient is applied to the skin, the DHA in the product reacts with the amino acid groups in the skin, supplied by perspiration and keratin. DHA doesn't penetrate the skin; the action of this chemically induced tan takes place on the stratum corneum, which is the outermost part of the skin, consisting of dead cells. The thickness and denseness of the stratum corneum of the skin determines the depth of the color. The face requires more frequent applications than the body. If the self-tan product is applied over areas that have rough, dry patches it will pick up the color unevenly.

THE PERFECT "SUNLESS" TAN—NO-FAIL WAYS TO ACHIEVE A DEEP, DARK TROPICAL TAN

Different self-tan products for different skin types: You may need to use two different types of self-tan products: a lighter consistency for the face and one that is richer for your body. There are quite a few companies that offer self-tan products according to your skin type (normal-to-dry and normal-to-oily).

Remove Dead Skin Cells and Moisturize

Before applying any self-tan product you should condition your skin. Plan to exfoliate and moisturize your skin at least one week in advance before using a self-tan product. Priming your skin is the key to achieving a natural-looking tan, and those few extra minutes a day of pampering will truly make a difference.

Gently buff the skin on your face with a fine facial scrub and use either a body scrub, exfoliating mitt, or loofah sponge on your body. Concentrate on areas that tend to get callused and rough such as the backs of arms, elbows, knees, and ankles. The object of this step is to remove the dead skin cells to create a satiny-smooth skin surface that will allow an even tan.

How to Prevent Your Sunless Tan from Fading

The active ingredient in self-tan products affect only the outer skin surface, which is made up of dead skin cells. As these cells shed or are sloughed off, your tan will fade. Reapplying your self-tan product frequently is necessary if you want to sustain your sunless glow.

Don't Have a False Sense of Security

Self-tan products are not a replacement for a sunscreen product, and the artificial tan won't protect you from UV radiation. Even if your sunless-tanning product contains sunscreen, the protection is usually worn off by the time you're out in the sun. For your own safety, use a sunscreen with an SPF of 15 or higher when outdoors.

Avoid Uneven Sunless Tanning

Don't apply self-tan products haphazardly because you can easily miss or streak an area. I guess the best way to describe the application of this product is to compare it to painting a wall. The first coat must be thin and even; I like to call this application the base coat. When this is completely dry, apply a second coat, which I call the finishing application. Pay close attention to the problem areas that tend to have a rougher, thicker texture such as the backs of arms, elbows, knees, and ankles because these areas seem to absorb more color and you don't want them to be darker than the rest of your body.

Incorporate Self-Tan Products into Your Skin-Care Routine

To incorporate self-tan products into your skin-care routine follow these steps:

1. Cleanse your skin.
2. Exfoliate.
3. Apply your self-tan product.
4. When the self-tan lotion is completely dry, apply your moisturizer.

Health Watch

If you use Retin-A medication, exercise caution when you use self-tan products. Because Retin-A affects the outer layer of the skin, it may cause your sunless tan to become uneven or to streak. But on the other hand, it may have no negative effect at all. In general, Retin-A and self-tan products are safe to use together, but you should adjust the amount of the self-tan product. Less is best. If your skin is a little on the dry and flaky side because of this medication, ask your physician if you can use an extra-fine facial scrub to buff away the flakiness and a water-based moisturizer to help with the dryness. Make sure you ask your doctor because you don't want to interfere with the Retin-A treatment.

The Don'ts of Self-Tanning Products

- Don't just slap this type of product on your skin. You must apply with even strokes.
- Don't apply a new self-tan product all over your face or body without first doing a small patch test on either your neck or under your chin. This will help you determine if the shade you've selected (light, medium, or dark) is appropriate for your skin tone. It is especially important to follow this advice when using this product on your face. It is always best to go with a lighter shade on the face if you have a fair complexion. Once you have established some color with the product you can graduate to a medium if you want to be darker.
- Applying lots of product doesn't give you a darker shade. Depth of color is achieved by layering applications over a period of several days.
- Don't apply self-tan products over dry, flaky skin because your sunless tan will look uneven in color. Exfoliate before using this product and moisturize your skin every day to help keep your skin from looking parched.
- Don't get dressed immediately after applying self-tan products. You should wait until your skin is completely dry, anywhere between 30 to 60 minutes. Also watch what you rub your skin against while the product is still moist because you might stain fabric and light-colored furniture.
- Don't use a self-tan product on acne skin because it will just accentuate the problem with uneven color. If you happen to have a few blemishes, you shouldn't have a problem. If you're using blemish medication, apply it approximately 2 1/2 hours after applying the self-tan product.
- Don't cover your lips, eye area, and ears with self-tan products. Blend the self-tan up to the lip line and go no further. Avoid your eyelids, brow bone and inner ears. To create a natural look on your ears, just blend a little product to the outer ear rim.

SUM IT UP!

How effectively you protect yourself and your family's skin from the sun or from tanning booths can influence your health and the way your complexion will look in years to come; it can also prevent skin cancer. Applying a maximum-strength sunscreen with an SPF of 15 or higher every day should be a way of life just like brushing your teeth or washing your hands. Please take the information in this chapter seriously and follow the advice of the American Academy of Dermatology because the sun truly is the cause of damaged and prematurely aged skin. So if you want to lessen your chance of skin cancer as well as maintain a youthful appearance or if you do not want to accumulate any more sun damage, avoid unprotected exposure to the sun as if it were poison.

CHAPTER *Eleven*

BEAUTY ON THE ROAD MADE SIMPLE

Caring for your skin doesn't have to stop when you are on the road for either business or pleasure. You say you don't want to lug around a cosmetic case that weighs 50 pounds? Well, beauty on the road can be simple, and your supply case should be as light as a feather. The following tips can help you survive the "skin nasties" of traveling.

Come on now, I know we are all guilty of packing a little too much. To prevent this from happening you should have various size kits for different time frames of travel. When I used to travel, anxiety would set in when it came time to pack my toiletry bag. Grabbing everything in sight, I would compulsively shove all this beauty stuff into a small carry-on bag. It was so full I had a hard time zippering it, but I was determined to be prepared for anything. Unfortunately, all those little lightweight bottles and jars collectively added up to the heaviest small bag in history. And the funny thing was that I didn't touch half of the stuff I packed. Soon I learned that traveling is stressful enough without the added pressure of being a pack mule. Now I'm proud to say I have broken this impractical habit and have became a most efficient traveler. I've learned that even the most comprehensive collection of travel products, accessories, and toiletries should weigh no more than 12 to 16 ounces—that's lighter than a pair of shoes, and I don't mean combat boots.

ANTI-STRESS ALERT—ANXIETY-FREE PACKING MADE EASY

Don't even think about bringing your full-size skin-care, hair-care, or nail products. The trick to this whole adventure is to minimize the weight of an item by giving yourself an appropriate portion. For example, you would never finish a six-ounce cleanser in a weeklong trip; that's probably a six-week supply. This holds true with all your products. Beauty on the road doesn't have to be compromised, and it doesn't mean that you will be stranded with just your toothbrush, toothpaste, deodorant, and a tube of moisturizer because you want to travel light. The following information will help guide you in organizing your packing.

The trick to anxiety-free packing is to have three plastic-lined cosmetic bags that zipper, plus plenty of empty travel-size bottles and jars. Two of the bags should be purse size and one should be large. The price for these bags ranges between $5 and $15. Empty travel-size bottles and jars are an important part of organizing your beauty supplies for traveling. All these items can be found in most department stores, discount stores, and large pharmacies, and they are worth every penny.

Step One: Purchase Three Skin-Care Cosmetic Bags

Bag 1 Purse-size, holds: cosmetics, nail care, toiletries, perfume

Bag 2 Purse-size, holds: prescriptions, over-the-counter remedies

Bag 3 Large-size, holds: skin-care and hair-care supplies

Step Two: Purchase Empty Bottles and Jars and Transfer Product Make a list of the skin-care, body-care, hair-care, and makeup products you want to transfer into smaller containers. The approximate unit cost for the empty packaging is usually under a dollar.

To keep your products clean, you shouldn't use your fingers to transfer the product. Use a small spatula or a butter knife to transfer the products into the alternative travel-size packaging.

If you have any doubts about quantities and you're tempted to bring extra, review the portion-control guide in Chapter Three; it will bring you back to reality.

DAILY ESSENTIALS FOR YOUR SKIN—THE SIX-OUNCE BEAUTY SURVIVAL BAG

This bag is so light that you should use it every day to hold your cosmetics and the little extras in your purse. It should weigh approximately six ounces.

Cosmetics, Toiletries, Nail Care, and Perfume

Foundation (1/4 ounce jar*)

Small translucent powder (1/4 ounce jar*)

Eye shadow and small brushes

Mascara

Lip pencil and lipstick

Small blush with a retractable blush brush

Travel-sized toothbrush and toothpaste

Emery board, smooth buffing nail file, nonacetone nail wipes **

Cuticle nipper, mini-size nail polish, and clear top coat

Hand creme (travel size—1/4 ounce)

Premoistened anti-microbial cleansing wipes for the hands (travel size—.006 ounce)

Deodorant

Atomizer (1/4 ounce of your favorite perfume)

MEDICINE ALERT—ONE SMALL TRAVEL BAG THAT WILL PREPARE YOU FOR A CRISIS

This bag can also become part of your everyday supplies that you bring with you to the office. You will always be prepared.

Prescriptions and Over-the-Counter Remedies When you pack over-the-counter remedies, if at all possible try not to use liquid

---

*You must transfer your foundation and powder from their full-size packaging into small travel jars.

**Nonacetone nail wipes are prepackaged towelettes. They will remove your nail polish, and they won't leak in your purse or suitcase.

products. Try the ones packaged as tablets, pills, or capsules. They are much lighter, and they won't leak. Always keep this bag in your purse, briefcase, or carry-on bag when you travel. This will reduce the chance of your misplacing or losing your prescription medication.

BEAUTY BASICS IN A BAG—YOUR SKIN, HAIR, AND NAILS WILL THANK YOU

The great thing about this bag is that once you get it organized it will always be ready for you. All you have to do is replenish the products you used on the trip and you will be ready for your next excursion. Just keep this bag in a cool, dry place in one of your closets.

Skin Care and Hair Care for the Two or Three Day Trip

Cleanser	1 ounce jar
Toner	1 ounce bottle
Moisturizer	1 ounce jar
Night creme	1/2 ounce jar (only if it is part of your routine)
Body lotion	2 ounce bottle
Sunscreen	travel size (if you are vacationing for a week or longer use a larger size)
Shampoo	2 ounce bottle
Hair conditioner	1 ounce jar
Hair spray	small travel size (approximately 1/4 ounce)
Styling gel or mousse	1/4 ounce jar

Accessories

Textured cleansing sponge

Headband

Cotton pads

Small, lightweight blow dryer

Brush and comb

THE LITTLE EXTRAS THAT WILL COMFORT YOUR SKIN WHEN YOU TRAVEL

If you are traveling for more than seven days you have the option of adding the following items to the bag:

- 1/4 ounce facial scrub
- 1/4 ounce masque
- 1/8 ounce eye creme

If your skin needs any special products such as an acne product or an AHA product, don't forget to bring them along, but be sure to transfer them into a smaller package.

EIGHT SURVIVAL TIPS FOR THE WEARY TRAVELER

Hours of plane travel can leave you a bit dehydrated. Drink plenty of water the day before and after your plane excursion. On the plane sip plenty of mineral water, seltzer, or plain water. Tea and coffee do not count because they act as a diuretic. Nibble on plenty of fresh vegetables and fruit.

Mist your face frequently with mineral water or alcohol-free toner that you have placed in a small purse-sized atomizer. It's refreshing, soothing, and it will help rehydrate your skin. And if you want a special treat, add a few drops of essential oil to the water in the atomizer—lavender to calm or lemon to refresh.

A day of traveling on a plane, train, or automobile can make you feel disheveled and frazzled. Want to look your best when you arrive at your destination? Get out your small cosmetic bag filled with all those beautifying goodies. Follow the next few steps and you will feel like a new person in less than three minutes:

1. Mist your face with the atomizer filled with water.
2. Apply a dab of foundation right over your make-up and dust it with translucent powder.
3. Cleanse your hands with the premoistened towelettes and apply your hand creme.

4. Give yourself a spritz with your purse-sized atomizer. You're as good as new!

Is tension building because of delays? A small drop of peppermint oil that has been preblended with a base oil (there are many prepared products sold in salons, bath stores, and department stores) massaged into each temple as you close your eyes for a minute or two will help you diffuse your tension and give you a moment of well-deserved peace.

Are your feet tired and overheated? Just spray your atomizer filled with water and a few drops of either lavender or lemon essential oils or freshener right through your stockings. It dries instantly and will cool off your feet every time.

Does your hotel or motel room ever have a stale odor? Did you know that if you light a small scented candle (takes up very little room in the suitcase) the air in your room will freshen up in no time. A few drops of your favorite essential oil will also do the trick.

Skin can become stressed out on the road. Don't hesitate to give yourself an exfoliating and masque treatment. Put your feet up on a pillow while the masque is setting.

The air can be drying in planes and hotel rooms. A little extra moisturizer may be necessary. After you have applied your moisturizer, if your skin still feels tight, apply a second application of moisturizer to counteract the extra dryness.

Are you the type of person who seems destined to develop a pimple or two when you travel? If you want to quickly soothe a large, conspicuous pimple, apply an ice cube directly on the blemish. It will reduce the inflammation.

SUM IT UP!

Traveling offers many challenges, so it's always important to have a few skin-care survival tips up your sleeve. The key to eliminating unnecessary frustration and anxiety is to be organized in your packing so you don't forget anything. Create a list of your toiletry and medication needs and decide how you're going to pack them; this is the route toward anxiety-free traveling. If you utilize this simple-to-follow, convenient, lightweight and economical travel plan, you will become a well-seasoned packing expert.

Part THREE

Professional Care

CHAPTER *Twelve*

MEDICAL UPDATE! DERMATOLOGY AND COSMETIC SURGERY OPTIONS

Your face represents your identity, so when you develop a skin problem it can strike a direct blow to your self-esteem. You may feel great emotional distress if you are experiencing a skin disorder, a skin disease, scarring due to chronic acne or an accident, or signs of premature aging due to sun damage. These are all reasons why you may want to seek the help of a medical specialist. Whatever your reason for seeking medical guidance, there are a whole realm of effective dermatologic or cosmetic surgery options available today that can correct or control skin problems or disfigurements. Medical treatments come in many forms such as topical creams and ointments, oral prescription drugs, chemical peels, or even cosmetic surgery.

In this chapter you will discover a wealth of up-to-date facts on the latest dermatologic procedures for treating acne and sun-damaged skin. You will learn what you can expect from skin lightening, Retin-A treatments, chemical peels, dermabrasion, laser procedures, and collagen injections.

Also, you will discover the many different types of cosmetic surgery that can help soften the signs of aging. You will find answers to questions like: "What is the appropriate age to consider a face lift?" "What can you expect from liposuction?" "How will I feel after a chin augmentation?" "How can I find a qualified cosmetic surgeon?"

THE STRAIGHT TALK ABOUT ACNE THAT WILL CLEAN UP ANY MISCONCEPTIONS YOU MAY HAVE

There are two main types of acne: noninflammatory and inflammatory. Noninflammatory acne consists basically of blackheads and whiteheads. This type usually results from clogged pores that have filled up with sebum and cellular debris. When this type of lesion has a covering or sac on top of it, it is called a closed comedone or whitehead. When the pore becomes filled with sebum and dilates, it is called an open comedone or blackhead. Blackheads are not filled with dirt, so you can't get rid of them by scrubbing. The dark color of the blackhead is caused by the accumulation of melanin cells and by an oxidation process that occurs when the solidified sebum comes in contact with the air. These noninflammatory lesions are the precursor of the inflamed lesions.

Inflammatory acne is divided into two categories: early inflamed (papule and pustules) and more severely inflamed (cysts and nodules). If a simple, noninflamed whitehead ruptures under the surface of the skin, it triggers an involuntary response that sends inflammatory cells to the site. Sometimes bacteria will grow on the sebum that has leaked from the pimple into the surrounding area. Once this chain of events has taken place, a noninflamed pimple becomes an inflamed pimple or pustule. This situation can also transform a simple pimple into a more solid type of lesion under the surface of the skin, called a cyst. Cysts are also commonly referred to as "underground" or "blind" pimples. They often seem to pop up overnight on the chin area, especially in women who are premenstrual. This type of pimple is usually surrounded by a great deal of inflammation, bacteria, and sebum. This combination of substances develops into a ball-like bump under the skin that can become tender or painful. If the cyst progresses in size and becomes more inflamed, it is referred to as a nodule.

REVEALING AN OLD ACNE MYTH THAT WILL ELIMINATE EMBARRASSMENT

Many individuals think acne is caused by dirt. They believe that if they scrub their face and clean it over and over again, the acne will improve. Actually that type of treatment backfires. If you over-cleanse the area, you strip the surface oils from the skin and you might actually stimulate the sebaceous (oil) glands to produce more oil (sebum) to help compensate for overwashing. Ultimately you can worsen the acne condition.

Dr. Diane Berson, assistant clinical professor of dermatology at New York University Medical Center, says that simple clogged pores can be kept under control if they are washed with an over-the-counter product that contains salicylic acid. If you have oily skin and clogged pores, this topical treatment can effectively unclog the pores. If you have a few lesions (pimples) that are in the very early phase of inflammation you might use an over-the-counter strength benzoyl peroxide medication to dry up the pimple. Benzoyl peroxide also acts as a powerful anti-bacterial agent, especially in prescription strength. But if you do not respond to these over-the-counter topical acne treatments, you should seek a dermatologist's care before the acne problem gets out of hand and causes permanent scarring.

Treating Mild Acne

There is a variety of medical treatments for mild acne—from topical creams and ointments to oral antibiotics; from extra-strength topical benzoyl peroxides to Retin-A or Accutane. When you have very small inflamed lesions (pimples) you may respond well to prescription-strength topical medications. When there are more inflamed lesions or when you have the cyst-type acne, then it is usually necessary to add an oral antibiotic (tetracycline, erythromycin, minocycline, or clindamycin) therapy to the acne regimen.

Self-Induced Acne Scars

You should not self-treat your acne (no matter what kind you have) by squeezing or picking the pimples or cysts. This can multiply your acne problem tenfold. Squeezing and picking can trigger a chain reaction because you are causing the lesion (pimple) to rupture under the surface of the skin. What follows isn't pleasant because you have increased the inflammation and have possibly caused a permanent scar. You can also turn that innocent little pimple into a painful underground cyst.

Physicians can correctly remove blackheads and whiteheads with a sterilized implement called an extractor. The dermatologist might even inject the cyst with an anti-inflammatory agent to shrink it. But if you do your own extracting with your unsterilized fingernails you will make the situation worse. Although very tempting, it is better to follow the hands-off policy.

Treating the Most Severe Type of Acne

If cystic acne is left untreated it can cause severe scarring—the most dramatic type being what's called the "ice pick" scar. In the past a person who had cystic acne didn't have many treatment options beyond oral antibiotics. Once someone developed cysts, they developed lasting scars. These scars are very difficult to rectify: collagen injections don't work very well, and although dermabrasion might help a little, it may not get rid of the scarring completely.

Fortunately, the next generation will not see this type of severe scarring as often because of a prescription drug call Accutane. Accutane is an effective prescription, topical medication—but it is not for everyone. Dr. Berson says you must know the contraindications before you use it: You can't get pregnant while you're on this drug; you cannot have liver disease; you can't have high cholesterol and triglycerides; you have to be aware that your skin and eyes will become extremely dry. Dermatologists monitor their Accutane patients very carefully. Dr. Berson sees these patients every month, and she gives them a blood test to monitor liver function, cholesterol and triglyceride levels, and if appropriate, she will administer a pregnancy test. Dr. Berson feels that Accutane is a safe therapy when patients are aggressively monitored.

Severe cystic acne or adult acne can also be treated with systemic prescription drugs such as oral antibiotics. And if the cysts get out of control, an anti-inflammatory cortisone drug can be injected directly into the cyst to shrink it, giving a better cosmetic appearance and making the cyst less itchy and painful.

Oral Antibiotics

Oral antibiotics are used to treat acne because they are both antibacterial and anti-inflammatory. They are often more effective than topical acne treatments on certain forms of inflamed acne for several reasons: Using a topical drying agent isn't going to be enough if you have a three-dimensional pimple. (You know the type if you have one; it looks and feels like a small ball.) A drying creme may help a little but it won't penetrate into the inside of that lesion. In this situation you need something internal that will go through the blood stream to get inside this type of cystic lesion. That's why your dermatologist may add an oral treatment to your regime if you don't respond to a topical agent.

When Can You Expect Results from Your Acne Treatment?

Dermatologist Berson doesn't want her acne patients to have any misconceptions when they begin their acne therapy so she tells them right away that their acne won't clear up overnight. If you don't have an accurate or realistic view about when you will see results, you may feel disappointed and frustrated and give up the treatment. The best advice to anyone being treated for acne is to be patient and stick with the treatment. Eventually you will see results.

You might see a little improvement after one full month of treatment. But depending on how severe the acne is, it usually takes anywhere from three to six months before you see a dramatic improvement.

Acne Maintenance

You must continue medical treatments until your skin is completely clear of the acne. Then, if you are still "acne prone," the next phase of the acne treatment, called acne maintenance therapy, will begin. This therapy will keep the pores unclogged and prevent the possible development of new inflamed lesions (pimples). This preventive treatment is extremely important. Retin-A has been used as an acne maintenance treatment because it helps to unclog the pores, preventing comedones (blackheads and whiteheads) from forming in the first place. As a maintenance treatment, Retin-A can help arrest the development of acne in its very early stages. Retin-A is also used to shrink blackheads and whiteheads making them loose and easier for your dermatologist to extract.

Adult Acne

Classic acne is characterized by basic clogged pores, blackheads, and whiteheads caused by oily skin. When puberty kicks in you begin to see more of the inflamed type of pimples: the papules and pustules. These new eruptions are due to the surge of hormones during this stage of life. When hormones fluctuate again in later life (especially when women are premenstrual, premenopausal, or pregnant), acne may again appear. Unlike teenage acne, which usually appears on the forehead, upper cheeks, and nose, the cysts of adult acne are usually found on the lower half of the face: the lower cheeks, jawline, the chin, and the upper neck.

Stress and Adult Acne

Stress is another catalyst that can trigger an acne flare-up because the body responds to the crisis by secreting a surge of hormones (androgens). Stress can cause the same kind of cystic acne you may experience when you're premenstrual, premenopausal, or pregnant.

How Dermatologists Treat Adult Acne Complicated by Sun Damage

Dr. Berson believes that glycolic acid is an appropriate therapy in the treatment of acne that is complicated by sun damage. Glycolic acid is an alpha hydroxy acid (AHA), which helps unclog the pores and therefore helps prevent an acne breakout. AHAs also exfoliate the outermost layer of the skin (stratum corneum), which, when sun damaged, can be dry, dull, and rough looking. By shedding the dead skin cells you achieve a much smoother-textured, more even-toned skin. This therapy can even remove some precancerous cells or early sun-damaged cells. There are plenty of over-the-counter AHA products that can work in combination with other acne treatments but you shouldn't self-prescribe your treatments. Never mix your treatments without consulting with a dermatologist, even if it is a nonprescription form of glycolic acid.

Daily Care for Acne Skin

When you are being treated for acne your skin may become very dry, making it more susceptible to skin sensitivities. It is important to use a mild, oil-free cleanser and moisturizer on the dry areas. To avoid unnecessary burning or irritation you should also use fragrance-free products.

UNCOVER A WHOLE NEW LAYER OF SMOOTH YOUNG SKIN

There are three characteristics of your skin that can be improved: texture, tone, and three-dimensional appearance. These improvements can be achieved with one or a combination of the many medical treatments available today in the form of prescription-strength topical and oral medications, and with several surgical procedures. Individuals with skin problems due to either acne scars, surface scars from an accident, sun damage, or aging have a chance to enhance the appearance of the skin with professional dermatologic care. Skin tone and three-dimensional changes can be achieved with cosmetic surgery (information about this option begins on page 299 of this chapter). This next section will address the use of Retin-A, hydroquinone (skin lightener), alpha hydroxy acids (AHAs), chemical peels, dermabrasions, and collagen injections.

RXS THAT WILL SMOOTH AND LIGHTEN YEARS OFF YOUR COMPLEXION

Retin-A/Retinoic Acid

A derivative of vitamin A, retinoic acid (also known as Tretinoin-Retin-A) has been used for over 15 years as a treatment for acne. Topical application of retinoic acid can help freshen a complexion and reduce symptoms of sun damage. This prescription drug can also lessen pigmentation problems associated with aging, make wrinkles and fine lines less visible, and speed cellular turnover.

You may need to apply this topical medication for two or three months or longer before you see a renewed glow in your complexion. Other changes in the skin's surface texture may take up to five months to become evident. Many dermatologists feel that retinoic acid treatments must continue for a lifetime to maintain the results. Others believe the skin needs an occasional rest from the drug. But all agree that this type of treatment is long-term.

When using retinoic acid, you will need to adjust your skin-care products and beauty routine because retinoic acid thins the stratum corneum, making your skin more sensitive. Switch to a milder, fragrance-free cleanser and moisturizer; use an alcohol-free toner.

Any time you use retinoic acid, wear a maximum-strength sunscreen because your skin will be photosensitive. If you do experience unprotected sun exposure while using this drug, you may develop pigmentation disorders, uneven skin tones and blotchiness, as well as burnlike inflammation.

The potential side effects of retinoic acid range from peeling, mild irritation, and redness, to extreme irritation. Your dermatologist will select the appropriate dosage and regimen based on your type of skin.

Hydroquinone

Hydroquinone is the active ingredient used in bleaching cremes. These cremes affect the skin superficially to lighten both abnormal and normal pigmentation. The effectiveness of the product depends on the individual and the severity of the problem. Many pigmentation problems (such as sun spots, age spots, liver spots, and freckles) are caused by being exposed to the sun's UV rays over a period of time without sunscreen protection. Hydroquinone depigments the skin, bleaching the increased melanin (color of the skin) that sometimes appears in cases of pregnancy mask and with the use of oral contraceptives.

Most dermatologists say that over-the-counter strengths of hydroquinone are ineffective, but that prescription-strength drugs can be highly effective. It is always best to consult with your dermatologist if you want to begin a skin-lightening treatment.

Alpha Hydroxy Acids (AHAs)

The leading ingredients in skin-care products today are alpha hydroxy acids. In the late seventies, dermatologists began using these ingredients; then lower strengths of the acids began appearing in over-the-counter products.

According to Dr. Harold J. Brody, clinical associate professor of dermatology at Emory University in Georgia, there are many types of alpha hydroxy acids. Two popular types are glycolic acid (derived from sugar cane) and lactic acid (derived from milk). These two acids are the AHAs with the smallest molecular size, which allows easy penetration of the skin.

While AHAs were originally derived from natural ingredients, today most are reproduced synthetically in labs. It is too costly and time consuming to create them any other way. Beta hydroxy acid has also been used in dermatology for some time. The only known beta hydroxy acid, to date, is salicylic acid, which is an ingredient used in acne medication and in foot-care products formulated to dissolve corns.

AHAs are in both over-the-counter and prescription medications. When you use over-the-counter-products containing AHAs, or when you get a nonmedical, salon peel (also called a "wash") containing AHAs, you are exfoliating the top dead layer of skin cells only. These over-the-counter AHA cremes can be used in conjunction with medical peels or nonmedical AHA washes. When a stronger prescription-strength AHA is applied by a dermatologist and the living layer of skin is affected, this is called a chemical peel.

COLLAGEN INJECTIONS

This medical procedure injects purified collagen (derived from animals) under the skin to help smooth wrinkles by filling the area directly under the wrinkle with collagen. (This helps plump the area.) This procedure is sometimes used for the more shallow type of acne scar to help elevate the area. How many injections you will need depends on how deep the wrinkle is and where it is located on your face. Collagen injections do not help all kinds of wrinkles such as deep lines on the forehead, for example. The type of wrinkles it does help are the kind that occur due to natural facial movements (frowning and smiling) around the mouth, nose, and eye area (such as crow's feet). The effects of this procedure should last anywhere between 6 and 18 months. This is a temporary treatment only and usually has to be repeated.

After having collagen injections, the skin at the injection site may look slightly bruised and may appear pink, but this will disappear in a few days. Also, the area may appear to look slightly raised, like a small bump, but this should gradually diminish (although there are some cases where the bumps may persist). If you are interested in collagen injections you should always be tested to see if you have any allergies to collagen. Also, anyone who has a history of rheumatoid arthritis or immunological disorders is not a good candidate for this procedure.

PEELING AWAY THE OLD SKIN TO REVEAL A NEW, PERFECT COMPLEXION

Various peeling agents have been used by the dermatology community for over 100 years. Because a large percentage of today's population is maturing and looking for treatments that can rejuvenate the skin, this well-seasoned medical treatment has resurfaced in the nineties. Chemical peels may not turn back the hands of time or stop the aging process, but they can soften the effects of aging, sun damage, and skin-surface imperfections, creating a fresher, more youthful skin surface.

What Can You Expect from a Chemical Peel?

Some of the conditions that respond well to chemical peels are fine wrinkles, sun-damaged skin (precancerous keratoses and scaly patches), mild acne scars, and irregular pigmentation (sun spots, age spots, liver spots, freckles, and blotchiness caused by oral contraceptives). Chemical peels cannot correct large pores, sagging skin, deep scarring, or dilated blood vessels on the face.

You will not see miraculous results overnight after one mild peel; it may take several peelings before you see the desired results.

For some conditions you may have to get a series of a half dozen to a dozen peels performed over a period of several months.

How Does a Chemical Peel Work?

Most medical peels involve the application of a mild peeling agent called trichloroacetic acid (TCA). This acid, used alone or with carbon dioxide or resorcinol, dissolves the uppermost layer of the skin. The chemicals "burn" the skin in a controlled manner (also known as chemical exfoliation), stimulating the growth of new, fresh, and improved skin. These mild peels are sometimes appropriately called "freshening peels," as are mild, new alpha hydroxy acid (AHA) peels. For some patients who may require deeper chemical peels, the chemical phenol is used. After a careful evaluation of the patient's condition, the dermatologic surgeon decides which agent should be used on what portions of the face or body.

How Will Your Skin Feel During Your Peel?

You will prepare for this procedure by protecting your eyes and hair, and your skin will be cleansed with a special agent to remove the surface oils. Once the chemical peel is applied, a warm-to-somewhat-hot sensation will be felt for about 5 to 10 minutes. Because the stronger medium-to-deep peels penetrate the dermis, pain medication may be given to avoid discomfort.

What Is the Recovery Time?

Because a chemical peel induces a controlled "burn" on the surface of your skin, your skin will look pink to red in color, depending on the strength of the peel. You might say it looks somewhat like a mild-to-severe sunburn.

"Dermatologists recognized the therapeutic benefits of chemical peeling as far back as 1903," says Dr. Brody. In 1984, 24 percent of the members of the American Academy of Dermatology reported that they were performing TCA face peels; 7 percent were performing phenol peels, and about 8 percent were performing more superficial peels. Dr. Brody believes these numbers have increased and perhaps even doubled just in the past seven years.

DERMABRASION! SMOOTHING AWAY THE OLD SKIN

"Dermabrasion is the dermatologic surgeon's most versatile modality to resurface and recontour the skin successfully," says Dr. Yarborough, clinical professor of dermatology at Tulane School of Medicine. Contemporary dermabrasion became popular in the 1950s with the introduction of the wire brush. The procedure has been refined, but the basic technique is essentially unchanged. Conditions that respond well to dermabrasion include recalcitrant acne, rosacea, dilated blood vessels on the face, actinic keratoses (precancerous lesions), sun-damaged and wrinkled skin, acne and chicken-pox scarring (combined with punch-scar elevation), accidental and surgical scars, freckles, and even tattoos. But dermabrasion is not effective in the presence of congenital skin defects, certain types of moles or pigmented birthmarks, or scars from burns.

Today, dermabrasion is performed using either a diamond fraise or a wire brush rotating at high speeds from power-driven instruments. These instruments are brushed across the skin (that has been frozen with cryogenic spray) to remove the top layer. General, regional block, or topical anesthesia can be used, depending on the physician's and patient's preference. This procedure, like chemexfoliation, is performed in the physician's office. The post-operative use of appropriate biosynthetic, semipermeable, or permeable membranous dressings has curtailed the need for narcotic analgesics to ease the discomfort.

Dermabrasion is highly regarded in the medical community. Dr. Yarborough reports that more than 12 years of follow-up evaluations of patients who underwent dermabrasion of sun-damaged skin confirmed the long-term, positive effects of this treatment.

Dermabrasion first gained attention for its treatment of acne scars. Since the mid-1970s, however, dermabrasion has been successfully used on small areas to obliterate or diminish facial lacerations following a biopsy, or accidental or surgical trauma. "If dermabrasion is performed four to eight weeks after injury, we have found that the scars will virtually disappear," says Dr. Yarborough.

It is important that any physician performing dermabrasion have extensive hands-on experience, and as with any surgical procedure, realistic expectations should be defined before both patient and physician mutually agree on the decision to operate. Dr. Yarborough feels that "this procedure should not be entered into lightly or without a complete understanding of the risks and benefits. The discomfort factor should be discussed openly and honestly. "But above all," he cautions, "be informed—ask questions!"

Questions to Ask Your Doctor About Chemical Peels and Dermabrasion

1. Considering skin type, skin color, age, medical history, and skin condition, am I a good candidate for a chemical peel or dermabrasion?
2. What are the risks of each procedure?
3. Are there any special prechemical peeling or predermabrasion procedures to be followed?
4. How long do I have to wear bandages after chemical peeling or dermabrasion?
5. How long will it take for my skin to heal after a chemical peel? After dermabrasion?
6. Which is better, chemical peeling or dermabrasion, to remove sun damage and wrinkles?
7. Should the skin be protected from the sun after chemical peeling and dermabrasion, and if so, for how long?
8. How long will a chemical peel or dermabrasion treatment last and what can be done to prolong its effects?

Conditions that Can Be Improved with Chemical Peels and Dermabrasion

Chemical Peels	Dermabrasion
Acne	Recalcitrant acne

Mild acne scars	Acne and chicken-pox scars (with punch elevation)
Sun-damaged skin	Sun-damaged and wrinkled skin
Fine wrinkles	Dilated blood vessels on the face
Lip-line wrinkles and crow's feet	Tattoo removal
Actinic keratoses (precancerous lesions)	Actinic keratoses (precancerous lesions)
Textural smoothing	Rosacea
Irregular pigmentation	Accidental and surgical scars
Freckles (lentigines)	Freckles (lentigines)
	Certain skin tumors
	Seborrheic keratoses (common growths on outer layer of the skin)

Disqualifying Conditions

If you have any one of the following conditions you would not be a good candidate for chemical peels and dermabrasion:

Chemical Peels	Dermabrasion
History of keloids	History of keloids
History of herpes simplex	History of herpes simplex
History of cardiac disease (deep peels only)	Burn scars
History of kidney or liver disease (deep peels only)	Giant hairy nevi (mole)
Previous facial radiation	Congenital skin defects
Recent isotretinoin treatment	Lentigo maligna
Recent isotretinoin treatment	Verrucae planae (flat warts)

BEYOND THE SCALPEL— BEAUTY ON THE CUTTING EDGE WITH BREAKTHROUGHS IN LASER SURGERY

Lasers have given a whole new dimension to surgical procedures. They have reduced risk of infection and given an alternative to the classic scalpel surgery. In some cases there is less scarring, and it is a relatively bloodless procedure. Lasers function by producing an intense beam of light that travels in one direction. The beam of light can cut, seal, and remove (vaporize) skin tissue and blood vessels in a relatively bloodless manner. Each laser will vary in intensity as well as in specific color; these two factors determine its application. There are a variety of lasers that are used in dermatology today, but there is no single laser that treats all skin conditions. The following information will give you a brief description of the most common forms of laser treatments.

The Carbon-Dioxide Laser (CO_2) (emits a colorless infrared light)

This laser is used in two ways: (1) for cutting the skin (surgical incision) and (2) to remove thin layers of the outer skin surface (soften the look of wrinkles) without cutting into deep layers. Warts, shallow tumors, and precancerous skin conditions of the lip can be treated with this laser.

The Argon Laser (emits blue and green light)

Elevated blood vessel growths, port-wine stain (purple-looking birthmark), enlarged blood vessels on the face, and the red-nose symptoms of acne rosacea can be treated by the Argon Laser.

The Yellow Light Lasers

The various yellow light lasers have been created to treat blood vessel conditions.

Argon-Pumped Tunable Dye Laser (emits a variety of colored lights)

A variety of blood vessel conditions are treated with this laser. It is also being used as an experimental treatment called Photodynamic Therapy for skin cancer.

Copper Vapor Laser (emits a green and yellow light)

The green light treats noncancerous brown-spot conditions like age spots. The yellow light treats blood vessel conditions like port-wine stain birthmarks and dilated capillaries.

Flashlamp-Pumped Pulsed Dye Laser (emits yellow light)

Port-wine stain birthmarks and dilated capillaries (telangiectasia) can be treated with the yellow beam of this laser.

The Ruby Laser (emits red light)

This was the first laser to be developed (created in 1959). Tattoos and brown spots from sun damage can be removed or faded with the ruby laser.

Coaxial-Flashlamp-Pumped Pulsed Dye Laser (emits green light)

This recently developed laser is used to treat a variety of brown-spot conditions such as old-age spots and sun-damage problems.

GET RID OF DEEP WRINKLES—ASTONISHING YOUTH-RESTORING COSMETIC SURGERY PROCEDURES

In today's society, there is an emphasis on achieving a healthy, youthful appearance. Often this is achieved through cosmetic surgery. The top 17 cosmetic surgery procedures performed in the United States in 1994 were liposuction, eyelid surgery, nose reshaping, chemical peels, hair transplant, face lift, dermabrasion, breast augmentation, chin augmentation, ear surgery, tummy tucks, breast reduction, breast lift, buttocks implants, buttock lift, calf implants, and pectoral implants.

The statistics are astounding. According to the American Academy of Cosmetic Surgery, 1,233,152 people had some sort of cosmetic surgery procedure in 1994 (914,676 females and 308,476 males). Although there are many reasons why individuals choose cosmetic surgery, certainly the end result is the same: a boost to self-confidence and self-esteem.

The work of a cosmetic surgeon requires not only medical skill, but artistic talent as well. With each procedure the body is sculpted to achieve improved contours. Cosmetic surgeons have the challenge of changing appearance, not only by affecting the texture of the skin, but also in a three-dimensional aspect. This type of surgery is often used to improve birth defects (example: cleft palate), permanent facial traumas (example: crushed cheekbone or chin due to a car accident), and scarring of the facial area and the body (example: deep lacerations). The field of cosmetic surgery makes daily, valuable contributions to the health of our society.

Improving Your Appearance with Cosmetic Surgery

Our skin constantly changes due to the abuse of unprotected sun exposure, the constant pressure of gravity, extreme fluctuations in weight, and the redistribution of fat cells and bone loss that occurs as we age. Some of these changes may make you think about having cosmetic surgery to regain a youthful appearance. There is no right or wrong choice when it comes to deciding whether or not to have cosmetic surgery. It's a private decision that is totally up to you—no one else should decide for you.

When making your decision, keep in mind that cosmetic surgery is not a cure-all. It won't solve any problems you are having in a relationship or at the office. And, you can't go to a cosmetic surgeon with a picture of a model and say you would like to have her nose. Think of cosmetic surgery as a tool to enhance your appearance, not totally change it. The surgeon has to work with what you have and make it all fit together.

The following descriptions supplied by the American Academy of Cosmetic Surgery will help you get a better idea of what to expect from some of the most popular cosmetic surgical procedures that are offered today.

BREAK THE TIME BARRIER— LEARN THE FACTS ABOUT COMPLETE FACIAL REJUVENATION

Aging is a natural process that frequently results in sagging and wrinkled facial skin. As we age, the muscles of the neck may also weaken. A cosmetic surgeon can help improve these conditions with a procedure called rhytidectomy.

The face lift (as we commonly call this procedure) "lifts" the face and neck. A "double chin" can be improved at the same time with a surgical procedure called submental lipectomy. Additional procedures, such as forehead lifting or eyelid surgery, can also be performed at this time for a more complete facial rejuvenation.

This type of surgery is requested by both men and women from as early as age 30 on into their seventies.

How Is a Face Lift Performed?

The incision for your face lift usually begins in the hair near the temple and continues along in front of the ear, around the ear lobe, behind the ear, and back into the hair. (This placement prevents easy detection.) The muscles and sagging tissues are tightened, excess skin is removed, and the remaining skin is repositioned to create a more youthful look.

If there is a double chin, submental lipectomy may be performed. A small incision is usually made under the chin so that the fat may be removed by liposuction.

The surgery takes an average of two to three hours and can be performed using either a local or general anesthetic. Preferences will be discussed with your cosmetic surgeon during your consultation. This operative procedure can be performed in the hospital or in an office surgical suite.

How Will I Look Immediately After the Surgery?

Some swelling and bruising should be expected; this normally subsides within several weeks. There may be some discomfort after the operation; this is usually controlled by medications prescribed by your cosmetic surgeon. Patients generally feel a sense of tightness and numbness that should gradually return to normal within several weeks. Sutures are usually removed approximately one week after surgery.

After recovery, you will have a more rested and youthful appearance. Although the positive effects of a face lift can last for many years, your skin will continue to age; therefore, it is impossible to predict how long it will be before you might consider a second lift.

What Are the Risks?

There are risks in any surgical procedure. Bleeding is the most common complication occurring occasionally after face-lift surgery. This can usually be treated without interfering with the final result. Occasionally, scars may have to be revised. You should discuss all the benefits and risks with your cosmetic surgeon.

EXTRAORDINARY EYES—REDUCE THE SIGNS OF AGING WITH THE LATEST SURGICAL TECHNIQUES

As we age, our eyelids undergo many changes that can make us look tired and older. Many factors, such as heredity and sun damage, accelerate these changes. Many younger patients will also complain of puffiness around the eyes, which can result from congenital changes leading to excess fatty tissue. Fat deposits, commonly called "bags," and loose skin of the upper and lower eyelids can be removed by your cosmetic surgeon in a procedure called blepharoplasty or "eyelift."

How Is an Eyelift Performed?

An eyelift can be performed on the upper or lower eyelids separately or both at the same time. The upper eyelid incision is made in the natural skin fold. The lower eyelid incision may be made directly under the eyelash line or on the inside of the lower lid. The excess skin and fatty tissue is removed and the incisions are carefully closed. The external incisions blend in beautifully and are virtually unnoticeable after a short time.

Blepharoplasty is commonly combined with a face or forehead lift as part of an overall facial rejuvenation. It can also be combined with chemical peeling to further enhance the results. Usually, a cosmetic surgeon will recommend the peel as a separate procedure, although it can be combined in certain situations.

This surgical procedure can be performed on an out-patient basis in the hospital, or in an ambulatory surgical suite under either general or local anesthesia, depending on the surgeon's and patient's preferences. When overhanging of the upper lids interferes with vision, the procedure may be covered by insurance.

How Will I Look Immediately After My Eye Lift?

Some swelling and bruising can be expected. The swelling will usually begin to subside within several days, while bruising may take several weeks to completely fade. Makeup can be used within a few days of surgery to cover any discoloration. Sutures are usually removed a few days after surgery. There may be mild discomfort after surgery that can easily be controlled by medications prescribed by your doctor. Generally, this procedure is well tolerated by patients.

What Are the Risks?

There are risks in any surgical procedure. You should certainly know that the degree of improvement varies from patient to patient. And you should discuss all the benefits and risks with your cosmetic surgeon.

DESIGNING THE PERFECT NOSE

There are many reasons people have cosmetic surgery performed on their nose. The nose may have an unattractive bump, or it may be too long or too wide. Cosmetic surgery can also rectify problems that contribute to breathing difficulties and headaches. Any or all of these conditions may be improved with a surgical procedure called rhinoplasty, or cosmetic nasal surgery.

During your initial consultation, the cosmetic surgeon will try to determine the changes you wish to make in your appearance. The surgeon will then help you understand the modifications that can be made and discuss any problems you may not be aware of. For example, many patients who seek rhinoplasty also have a very weak chin or flat cheekbones. In a case like this, chin or cheekbone implants might be considered as a part of the operative plan.

How Is It Done?

To begin rhinoplasty, the surgeon makes incisions inside the rim of the nostrils. Sometimes, tiny inconspicuous incisions are made on the rim of the nose. Soft tissues of the nose are then separated from the underlying structures. The cartilage and bone that are causing the external deformity are altered and reshaped. At the same time, internal problems, such as breathing obstructions, can be improved by removing the obstruction. This part of the procedure is called septoplasty.

Rhinoplasty and septoplasty usually take one to two hours depending on the amount of work that must be done. The procedure can be performed in the hospital or outpatient surgical suite. The surgery is commonly done under either local or general anesthesia, depending on patient and doctor preferences.

What to Expect During Recovery

To protect the nose during the first few days after surgery, a small cast or splint is placed on the nose and a light internal dressing may be applied. There will be some swelling and stuffiness for several weeks, but patients usually resume normal light activity after a few days. It will take several weeks before the nose is completely healed and you are allowed to resume full physical activity. Surprisingly, there is very little pain after rhinoplasty and most patients require only mild analgesics.

What Are the Risks?

Rhinoplasty will provide significant improvements in the vast majority of patients. But in occasional cases, a secondary correction may be required. Because there are risks in any surgical procedure, you should discuss all benefits and risks with your cosmetic surgeon.

NEW WAYS TO IMPROVE YOUR CHEEKBONES AND CHIN— THE POWER OF FACIAL IMPLANTS

Chin Augmentation

Many people have a chin that is too small for their face. This detracts from the overall appearance of the face and may also make the nose look larger than it really is. For this reason, many patients seek surgery to improve the shape of the chin. The operation can also greatly enhance the results of a face lift, since loss of chin projection may occur with aging. Chin augmentation is also commonly combined with facial liposuction, where fat is removed from under the chin and from the neck.

How Is a Chin Augmentation Performed? A small incision is made either underneath the chin or inside the mouth. A sterile implant, similar to the consistency of a natural chin, is placed in front of the chin bone to increase the projection of the chin. The implant is secured and the incision is sutured closed.

Cheekbone Augmentation High cheekbones are a sign of beauty. For those not born with this look, cheekbone augmentation may be the answer. The procedure consists of placing a synthetic implant over the natural cheekbone. Implants come in a variety of sizes and shapes so that the cosmetic surgeon can select the proper one for each patient. Men also frequently seek this operation to correct flatness in the mid-face. As is the case with chin augmentation, cheekbone augmentation is frequently combined with other cosmetic procedures such as rhinoplasty or face lift. Additionally, it is frequently combined with chin augmentation.

How Is a Cheekbone Augmentation Performed? A small incision is made inside the mouth in the crease above the upper lip. A sterile implant, similar to the consistency of the natural cheekbone is placed over the bone to increase its projection. The implant is secured and the incision is sutured closed.

These procedures can be performed with either a local or general anesthetic, depending on the preferences of the surgeon and patient. The operations can be performed in the hospital or in an outpatient surgical suite.

How Will I Look Immediately After an Implant?

Some swelling and bruising can be expected and usually subsides within the first two weeks. A tape of elastic dressing may be recommended for a period of time. Mild discomfort is usually easily controlled with medications prescribed by your cosmetic surgeon.

After healing, the skin drapes smoothly over the implants. The implants themselves conform to the bone and usually are undetectable. The added projection of the chin should result in significant improvement that is especially apparent in profile. The cheekbones can be expected to mimic natural high cheekbones.

What Are the Risks?

In rare circumstances, an implant may have to be removed or changed due to unexpected problems. This can usually be done with little difficulty. Occasionally, there may be temporary numbness after the surgery. There are risks in any surgical procedure. You should discuss all the benefits and risks with your cosmetic surgeon.

DISCOVER THE SECRET THAT WILL GET RID OF UNWANTED FAT CELLS

Many people have unwanted fatty deposits they can't get rid of with diet or exercise. These fatty deposits are commonly found in the areas of the thighs, hips, tummy, buttocks, waist, knees, and ankles. A procedure called liposuction removes these fatty deposits. Facial liposuction can also be performed to remove excess fat in the cheeks, jowls, neck, and chin areas. Facial liposuction can be carried out alone, or in combination with face lifting or chin augmentation.

How Is It Done?

The fatty deposits are suctioned out with a vacuum-type device. A tiny opening, usually 1/2 inch in length, is made in inconspicuous areas, through which a small tube or "cannula" is inserted. The tube is connected to a source of high suction and passed back and forth within the fatty tissue so that unwanted fat cells are loosened and suctioned away.

This surgical procedure can be performed on an out-patient basis in the hospital, or in an ambulatory surgical suite under either general or local anesthesia, depending on the preferences of the surgeon and patient. You will usually be required to wear a girdle or elastic neck strap (depending on location of the procedure) for several days following the procedure to provide support and to maintain your new shape. Most patients resume normal activity within a few days of the surgery.

How Will I Look Immediately After Liposuction?

Most patients experience bruising and swelling after liposuction that lasts a variable period of time. For that reason, it takes awhile before the final results of the surgery are apparent. However, the vast majority of patients are highly pleased with the results of liposuction surgery.

How Will I Feel After Liposuction?

Although discomfort is usually minimal, post-operative medications can be prescribed by your cosmetic surgeon to provide relief from any soreness. Many patients return to work within three to four days. There are usually very few restrictions on normal daily activities.

What Are the Risks?

Although no long-term adverse effects have been reported as a result of this procedure, there are risks in any surgical procedure. On rare occasions, some fluid accumulation may occur beneath the skin, and occasionally patients experience some numbness, which is usually temporary. Some irregularity of the skin may also occur, especially in patients with poor skin elasticity. You should discuss all the benefits and risks with your cosmetic surgeon.

What Is the Cost?

Fees for each procedure vary from one geographic area to another. For information on fees in your geographic area contact the American Academy of Cosmetic Surgery to request the current schedule of "Cosmetic Surgery Fees" (see Page 355).

SUM IT UP!

The way we look and how we perceive ourselves are at the root of our identity. The problem of skin disorders and diseases is a serious subject because it affects the largest organ of our body which is so visible for all to see. As you have learned in this chapter, today's medical options offer a variety of medications and surgical procedures that address the serious concerns and symptoms of skin cancer, acne, sun damage, aging, sagging facial skin and eyelids, fatty deposits, and unattractive nose, chin, or cheekbones.

The key to your medical skin treatment lies in locating a qualified dermatologist or cosmetic surgeon in your area. If you need assistance finding a physician, contact either The American Academy of Dermatology or The American Academy of Cosmetic Surgery (see Appendix A on page 351). These two national organizations can put you in touch with a qualified physician near you. There are plenty of professionals who can help control your skin problem or correct it, so if something about your skin or your appearance has been bothering you for a long time, maybe now is the time to look into changing the way you look with the help of a medical professional.

CHAPTER *Thirteen*

THE WONDERS AND TRUTHS OF PROFESSIONAL PAMPERING

The service industry of spas and salons has been around for centuries. Today there are many different types of facilities that perform professional skin-care treatments: there are skin-care clinics; medical offices; full-service salons that offer hair care, skin care, nail services, and makeup applications; day spas that offer an extensive menu of skin-care and body services in a serene atmosphere; and, finally, the full-service spa. It is this last skin-care facility that is the focus of this chapter.

There are nine different types of spas, but always there has been an air of mystery surrounding their beauty regimes and recipes. I thought it would be fun to give you an insider's look at some of the most renowned spas in the world and uncover their secrets. Let's find out how and why these highly trained professionals at international spas perform facials, eye treatments, neck and décolleté rejuvenation, algae body wraps, body mud packs, paraffin face and body treatments, thermal steam, aromatherapy hand and foot treatments, aromatic massages, sea salt and oil body treatments, glycolic acid face and body treatments, and on and on. Let's explore the hi-tech equipment they now use to reap the maximum benefits from natural elements such as sea water, algae, sea salt, ocean clay, essential oils, and ground loofah. Let's build mental pictures of how each one creates a retreat, an oasis, an escape that shields and protects guests from the outside world. We'll imagine the peaceful settings where the air is purified with the scent of delicate essential oils and the fragrance of fresh blossoms, where the decor is designed with soothing and delightful colors, artwork, and furniture, and where guests can disconnect from the busy world and enter a state of true peace.

WHAT KIND OF SPA ARE YOU LOOKING FOR?

There are nine different types of spas you can visit; each one caters to a special need. While you browse through their descriptions, keep an eye open for the one that best fits you; with their many affordable packages, spas are no longer for only the rich and famous.

The Fitness and Beauty Spa

This spa combines fitness and a touch of pampering. An eager staff of highly trained professionals will guide you on a path that will enhance your health and well-being. Your days will be filled with exciting fitness activities and delicious, nutritious food alternatives. After you work hard at reconditioning your body, you can take a pause and refresh yourself with a luxurious essential oils massage or a facial or body treatment. Your stay at the fitness spa will help you dissolve stress, unwind, and rediscover your true physical potential.

The Weight-Loss Spa

Here you will enter a supportive environment to start your journey toward a healthier body weight. Supervised medical care, diet changes, behavior-modification counseling, fitness coaching, and plenty of educational programs are at the heart of the weight-loss spa. Recognizing that the challenges of being overweight can be frustrating, the staff at this type of spa will help you set a more realistic approach to weight loss, designed for your special needs.

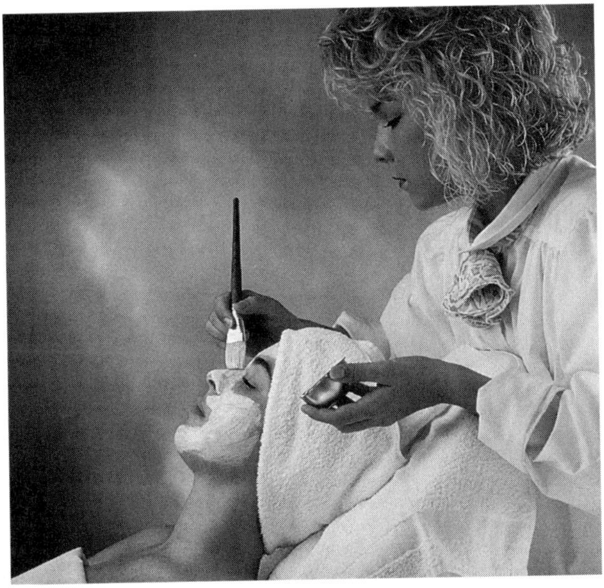

Canyon Ranch Health and Fitness Resort in Lenox, Massachusetts and Tucson, Arizona. Skin Softening Facial Masque Therapy.

The Resort and Spa

This type of spa can be found in the mountains, desert, forest, or by the ocean and can offer a diversity of amenities, including excellent hotel accommodations, sport activities (such as golf, tennis, and skiing), delightful dining experiences, entertainment, plenty of pampering spa treatments, and fitness activities. This mixed bag is perfect for people who want a flexible schedule—if you want to stay on the golf course all day or just escape into the spa to be massaged and pampered, the choice is yours.

The Luxury Spa

This spa offers red carpet treatment at its best! Every detail of your stay will be taken care of as if you were royalty. The luxury spa combines fine service with expert fitness advice, nutritional information, delicious low-fat meals, holistic beauty treatments, and massages. Here, you can have one-on-one consultations with personal fitness trainers, nutritionists, and beauty experts. All these activities take place in surroundings that are first-rate and serene. Nothing that contributes to your pampered pleasure is overlooked.

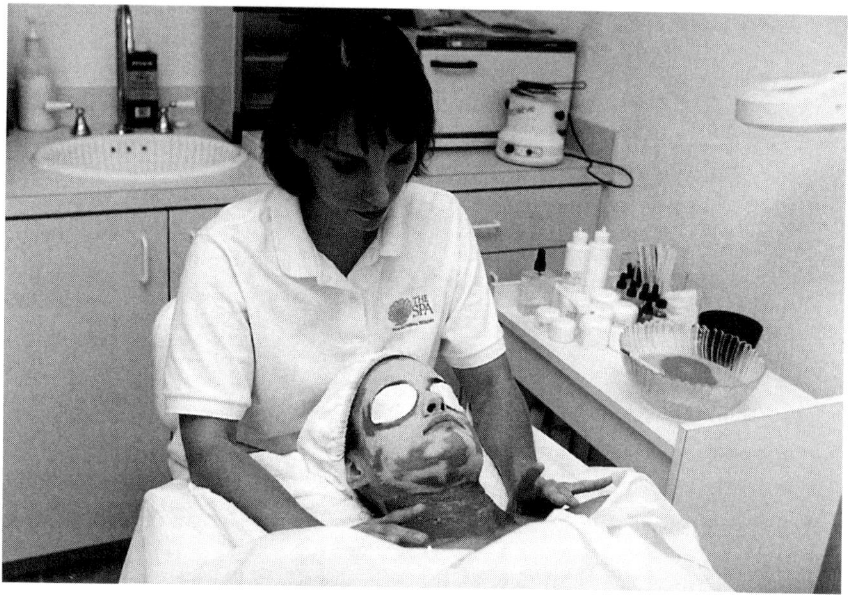

PGA National Resort & Spa, Palm Beach Gardens, Florida. Deep Cleansing Facial and Soothing Eye Compress.

The Mineral Springs Spa

At this spa, you will discover the most ancient and celebrated form of water therapy, better known as "taking the waters." A water experience is one of nature's most therapeutic treatments. Hot mineral springs from deep below the earth's surface are warm and rich in minerals and can be found in the United States and in Europe. Or, you can partake in what's known as thalassotherapy by soaking in purifying ocean mud, algae, or sea water. These forms of water therapy are not new—they were recommended by Hippocrates for their therapeutic benefits. Whether you choose mineral water, seawater, or the mineral-rich muds, you will feel stress melt away as your body becomes one with the warmth of the water surrounding your body.

The New Age Spa

Enter the world of alternative spas featuring holistic health and vegetarian eating and/or fasting. Experience ancient rituals and philosophies of meditation, yoga, astrology, deep relaxation, reflexology, and aromatherapy. New age sounds off the beaten path but this alternative to the classic spa is now quite popular.

Spa Abroad

Enhance your trip to Europe by staying at one of its world-class spas. The European spa and its approach to health, fitness, and beauty is renowned throughout the world (and is often imitated in many spas in the United States). Rest, relaxation, and the cure for ailments (under medical supervision) go hand in hand with the great mineral springs, the mineral-rich drinking water, and the opportunities for the application of mineral muds found throughout Europe.

The Adventure Spa

If you like excitement and physical challenges this type of spa is for you. Experience the wonders of nature as you explore and hike over the terrain: the Amazon jungle, the deserts and mountains of Utah, the mountains of New England, or the volcanos, jungles, and shore line of Hawaii. There are many locations to choose from, and the spa will provide an expert guide to lead you through the "great outdoors" safely. And don't worry—there are comforts and some pampering to look forward to also: massage, Jacuzzis, pools, and let's not forget the delectable spa cuisine.

The Floating Spa

Yes, you can visit a luxurious spa as you float on the sea in a majestic ocean liner. Explore the Mediterranean, Atlantic, Pacific, or Caribbean. Discover spa pleasures, relaxation, and beautifying treatments such as soothing facials, essential oil treatments, herbal wraps, and water treatments (hydrotherapy). Fine dining with healthful food choices and exercise classes with fitness experts will help you discover a new dimension in cruise vacations.

EXCLUSIVE AND LUXURIOUS SPAS IN AMERICA

There are so many four-star spas all over America that it is impossible to give you a peek inside them all. But here's a sampling of a few of my favorites to whet your appetite.

The Green Valley Spa, St. George, Utah

The State of Utah in the great American Southwest is a mecca of natural plants and minerals from the desert. The word *desert* implies a wasteland, but this is far from true when discussing the Mohave desert because it is bountiful in life, colors, and healthful mineral-rich salts, muds, and sands. The Green Valley Spa is extremely fortunate to be able to harvest the plant life, thermal muds, and mineral salts from this desert and use them in their treatments.

Carol Combs, owner of the spa, says they call the harvests of the desert "Good Medicine," which is a term used by the Indian Nations to describe anything that uplifts the spirit and brings pleasure and wholesome nourishment to body and mind. Carol states that she is indebted to our native predecessors (who inhabited this area as far back as 11,000 B.C.) for their understanding of the rich and beneficial plant life that graces her desert home. She calls upon their ancient knowledge to create the desert products and tinctures the spa uses in all its treatments. Plants like ephedra, alfalfa, and dandelion are very stimulating, juniper berries are germicidal, sage is clarifying, creosote contains purifying agents, aloe vera and potatoes are detoxifying, and yucca is cleansing. All are gathered from the desert next to the spa. The rainwater is captured as it falls through the clear desert air before it touches the soil. The rich essential minerals in the rainwater (that are not available in any other form) are mixed with the plants to create the treatments used in the spa.

A special treat at the Green Valley Spa are the mineral-salt therapies. This special bath additive contains noncultivated, untreated salts extracted from highly mineralized veins native to the red sandstone cliffs—once part of an ancient sea bed. These mineral salts are used to recreate the famous desert spring thermal waters revered for their soothing and rejuvenating virtues.

The wild beauty and mystery of the red-rock country surrounding the magnificent Green Valley Spa facilities offer the perfect environment to rekindle your energies. Their program of fresh air, exercise, nourishing food, quiet contemplation, and beautifying face and body treatments all contribute to a sense of well-being that pampers the spirits and energizes the body.

There are many individual spa services at Green Valley, but a few of the more unique ones include Full Body Canyonland Mud Pack, Crushed Pearl Body Rub, and Cinnamon Sugar Cellulite Treatments. Before every spa treatment the guests partake in a bath ritual that involves a prebath anointing with special skin-cleansing elements and rainwater from the desert, a bath in waters enriched with aromatic elements and mineral salts, and an after-bath moisturizing with desert oil essences. All treatment rooms have fresh flowers, aromatics, music, and scented water to tantalize and impress the senses.

Spa Grande at the Grande Wailea Resort, Wailea, Maui, Hawaii

Darryll Leiman of Spa Grande explains that this spa emphasizes traditional Hawaiian therapies using products from the region. "Just as regional cooking takes advantage of local flavors and raw materials," he says, "so Spa Grande offers beauty treatments that take advantage of regional Hawaiian therapies that have been passed down through generations using elements of the islands such as seaweed, Maui mud, ti leaves, sea salt, and algae clay." The following are some of the spa's special treatments.

Termè Wailea Hydrotherapy Water Circuit: The Termè Wailea Hydrotherapy Circuit includes a bath in a Roman hot tub and then a cool dip; then steam, sauna, Swiss jet shower, and Japanese furo tub. Add a cascading waterfall massage and a selection of essence baths such as the papaya enzyme and limu/seaweed baths and you are thoroughly rejuvenated.

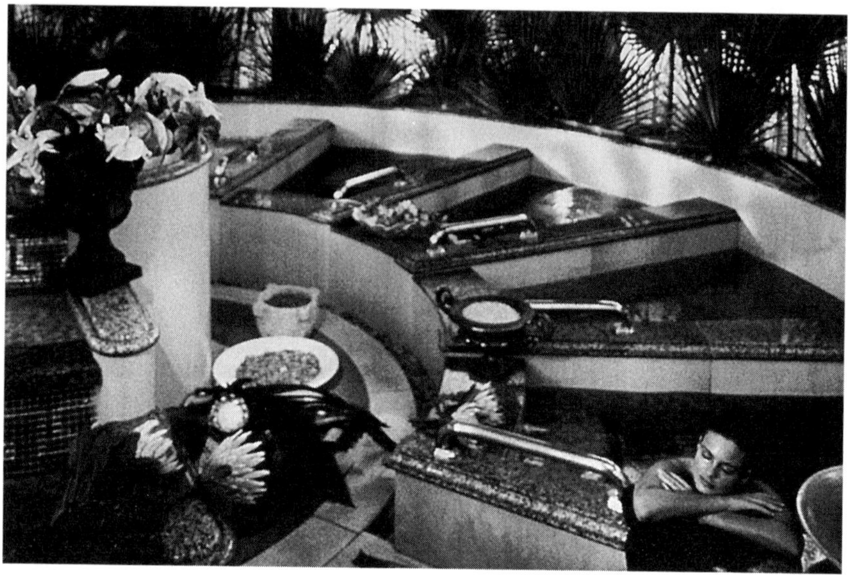

Spa Grande at the Grande Wailea Resort, Wailea, Maui, Hawaii. The Termè Wailea Hydrotherapy Circuit includes a Roman hot tob, and a cool dip, steam, sauna, Swiss jet shower, Japanese Furo tub, plus cascading waterfall and as shown the essence baths such as the papaya enzyme and Limu/seaweed baths.

Hawaiian Salt Glo: In ancient Hawaii, cleansing the body was a two-step process. First the body was "anointed" with oil and then (in lieu of soap) a mixture of clay, sand, and sea salt was used to exfoliate the skin. Today this ancient practice is repeated at Spa Grande with a mixture of Hawaiian red clay and sea salt, or fine Hawaiian sand as a gentle abrasive to remove dead skin and excess oils from the body. This also stimulates the circulatory system, which aids in the cure of afflictions. The skin is left feeling silky smooth, fresh, and vibrant.

Ali'i Honey Steam Wrap: Originating in Hungary and performed in various ways at spas in Germany and Italy, the Ali'i Honey Steam Wrap is one of the Spa Grande's "East meets West" treatments. "Ali'i" means royalty, and Spa Grande has taken highlights of this treatment and combined it with principles passed on by the Hawaiian kahunas. Using exclusively Hawaiian products, the treatment begins with a loofah scrub with honey mango bath gel, followed by further exfoliation with sea salt. Honey from the island of Molokai is then painted onto the body, followed by a linen wrap and a short stay in the steam room. The honey marinades into the skin, leaving it soft, vibrant, and tingling.

Hawaiian Limu Rejuvenator: This is a tension-relieving treatment. First, a masque made of limu seaweed is applied to the guest's back to detoxify the skin and absorb excess oils; then the body is massaged with aromatherapy oils using Lomi Lomi techniques.

Limu/Seaweed Bath: This therapy combines limu seaweed, mineral salts, kelp, and other plants from the seaweed family, agrimony (an herb from the rose family), and fragrance to create a warm, relaxing bath as opposed to a stimulating one. The seaweeds are vitamin and mineral rich, and act as a soothing emollient. Soaking in a bath of seaweed for 20 minutes will leave the skin and body refreshed. Combined with agrimony, it is an ideal treatment for tired muscles and joints.

Royal Hawaiian Facial: This treatment uses limu/seaweed to stimulate sluggish cells, eliminate toxins, and achieve a favorable balance for regeneration of cells. The facial begins with a relaxing heated hand and foot massage with papaya enzyme extract, followed by a deep cleansing, detoxifying facial, and a nourishing seaweed masque that purifies the skin while absorbing excessive oils, leaving the skin glowing with radiance.

Hawaiian Scalp Treatment: This relaxing therapeutic scalp treatment massages the scalp with enriching nutrients from the sea, along with essential oils. This is an ideal treatment for dry or dandruffed scalps.

Two Bunch Palms Resort and Spa, Desert Hot Springs, California

The ultimate pleasures at the Two Bunch Palms are the water and mud treatments. Millenniums ago, deep beneath the southern California desert, nature created one of the hottest artesian mineral wells in the world. The unparalleled water of this natural phenomenon shoots up from the deep double geological fault of Miracle Hill at approximately 148 degrees F. and then cascades downward to nurture the oasis of Two Bunch Palms.

In the warm mineral waters of this world-class resort and spa, guests enjoy Watsu under a grove of rustling palms. Watsu is short for "Water Shiatsu" which is more like passive yoga in water than massage. Some guests have described it as a return to the womb, where you hear your own heartbeat and become one with the water. Developed in the early 1980s by Harold Dull, director of Harbin's School of Shiatsu and Massage-Watsu, it is now practiced worldwide. Supported entirely by the water and a therapist, you are gently stretched and moved through the water, fluid and weightless. After Watsu, guests are refreshed and restored, often experiencing emotional release as the body responds. Because of the growing demand for couples Watsu, Two Bunch Palms has added its largest private pool, secluded beneath the rustling palms and warmed just below body temperature to 96 degrees F.

This pool also accommodates their newest hydrotherapy treatment, Wassertanzen (pronounced Vasser-tahn-sen). If Watsu is passive yoga, Wassertanzen is like passive ballet. This treatment starts as the therapist gently rocks and cradles you in the rejuvenating mineral water. As you unwind, the therapist guides you below the surface, where most of the body work occurs. The merger between above and below water is a harmonizing blend of timeless, weightless wonder. The underwater choreography distinguishes this treatment from all others. Developed in 1987 by Swiss trainers Arjana Brunschwiler and Aman Schroter, Wassertanzen has been described as the ultimate spa treatment. You learn to become seaweed floating in the currents of the water.

Nemacolin Woodlands Spa, Village of Farmington, Pennsylvania

The Woodlands Spa is nestled in the breathtaking vistas of the Laurel Mountains in Western Pennsylvania. Three stories and 20,000 square feet of architectural beauty and interior luxury are accented with antiques, artwork, marble floors, and cherry wood. One step into The Woodlands Spa and you are immersed in the exclusive tranquility of a world-class facility.

The therapeutic and aesthetic values of paraffin can be traced to ancient civilizations, states Kimberly Wright, body and beauty manager for the spa. The Romans poured hot oil and waxes on the body as a heat-inducing prelude to massage. The French brushed melted paraffin on wounds, while the British established paraffin as a modality for orthopedic disorders in the military hospitals of World War I. Today still, paraffin is embraced by the medical community and rehabilitation specialists for its therapeutic qualities. Now the spa industry is using its beneficial properties to treat its guests to a special regimen.

Paraffin therapy is a well-rounded thermotherapy. It reduces pain and stiffness around joints by assisting in the natural lubrication of surrounding tissue. Paraffin is especially beneficial in the treatment of arthritis, bursitis, tendonitis, overworked and fatigued muscles, and scar tissue that restricts range of motion in joints and tendons.

As a beauty treatment, the wax is layered onto the skin. An airtight seal is formed that introduces moisture into surface cells, plumping fine lines and moisturizing parched skin. This improves the texture, color, and general appearance of the skin.

Kimberly Wright describes a Full Body Paraffin Treatment at the Woodlands Spa. (This treatment should not be given to a person with diabetes, high blood pressure, heart problems, heavy varicose veins, open wounds, rashes, skin irritations, sunburn, windburn, claustrophobia, or to someone who is pregnant.)

Step One: Exfoliation With the guest lying on her stomach, the therapist uses a soft body brush to dry-brush the body, starting with the bottoms of the feet and moving upward to the legs, thighs, and back. This will help get rid of dry skin cells.

Step Two: Apply Moisturizer A body moisturizer is applied to the skin using long, relaxing movements.

Step Three: Paraffin Application Tissuelike towels are dipped into warm paraffin, then molded to the body. The spa guest is wrapped up with a mylar sheet and blanket to keep warm, relaxed, and comfortable for 10 minutes. The tissues are unwrapped and removed. The spa guest then turns over and the same treatment is repeated on the opposite side of the body.

Gurney's Inn Resort and Spa, Montauk, New York

The limitless therapeutic and beauty properties of seawater are well known at Gurney's International Health and Beauty Spa where beyond the bounty of wind-brushed bluffs spreads the undulating and cleansing ocean. Whether choosing the cool charge of an aquatic workout or the soothing sanctuary of a Finnish sauna, the concept of the spa is to restore perennial vibrancy. This spa has a sweeping selection of massage therapies to relieve tensions and fade fatigue, as well as other water therapies such as Swiss showers, Russian steam rooms, herbal wraps, fango packs, and seawater Roman Baths. In many forms, this spa taps into the benefits of seawater, which is scientifically proven to be the richest water of all, with many essential health-giving components. Our bodies contain almost the same amount of minerals found in seawater: calcium, potassium, and iodine along with other trace minerals, vitamins, and salts. That's why submerging in seawater makes you feel invigorated.

Seawater therapy is very popular at Gurney's. Tubs are filled with filtered ocean water and heated to body temperature. Relaxation is induced by underwater jets creating a gentle, floating effect. More powerful jet massage comes from six movable nozzles set into the tub's sides. A highly skilled therapist then manually water massages the body under the water with a special hose attachment. Afterwards, guests float peacefully on gentle water-powered currents.

The Spa Internazionale at Fisher Island Club, Fisher Island, Florida

This oasis of luxury is just a 10-minute ferry ride off the coast of Florida. At The Spa Internazionale guests experience the latest advancements in fitness programming, pampering, and invigorating body and skin-care treatments, all in a serene, tropical setting. The environment here simulates the soothing effects of the sea and sand with its color scheme of pale aqua and natural unstained ash.

A favorite beauty treatment of spa director Deborah Smith is the tension-relieving eye massage and mask. Nourishing AHAs (contained in ampules) and a special pressure-point massage drain away tension and relieve pressure in the sinus area. The use of the lymphatic drainage jet machine and the Lucas Championniere (a machine that projects water under pressure with an atomizer that diminishes the size of the fluid droplets that are dispersed onto the face) stimulates the skin with a soothing mist of lavender, cypress, geranium, thyme, or rosemary scent. This aromatic mist is then massaged into the skin. Then a gommage gel (containing carob bean, orange essential oil, lemon essential oil, sweet lime essential oil, and vegetable extracts) is applied to the eye area and is gently massaged to exfoliate the skin. The skin is then rehydrated with the aromatic mist of the Lucas spray. A blend of AHAs (alpha hydroxy acids) is applied to the eye area, and then the skin is gently buffed with a soft gauze. This procedure is repeated three times.

The skin is then massaged with three massage movements: Lymphatic, Shiatsu, and European. A custom-blended masque is then applied to the eye area. This special clay masque is mixed with a serum containing hops extract and a creme of rosemary extract. The masque is brushed around the eyes and a moist camomile tea bag is placed on each eye lid. While the masque is setting the guest can enjoy an accupressure massage on the feet. The masque is then removed with warm compresses and a moisturizer and eye creme are applied. This type of soothing treatment promotes whole-body relaxation as it refreshes the eyes and helps to reduce puffiness around the eyes.

The Sagamore Spa, An Omni Classic Resort On Lake George, Boltons Landing, New York

The Sagamore is nestled among the majestic mountains of the Adirondacks in New York State. The spa offers many unique face and body treatments but one of the msot unique concepts is the harvesting of Adirondack herbs and aromatic plants native to this mountain region. The main ingredients of the formulas have been used by native American tribes as part of their culture in terms of medicines and cooking. Early settlers learned how to use these herbs and barks to make teas and compresses to treat wounds and pains.

Pine and birch bark yield highly aromatic oils that leave a feeling of freshness while they help to improve oil secretions in the hair and scalp.

Marigold, chamomile, wintergreen, and peppermint are common to the area, also. Native Americans used these powerful herbs to calm stomach aches and help digestion. Topical applications of these beneficial plants helped especially to heal wounds and restore circulation to the skin.

Lastly, a pure concentration of wild chamomile, mountain thyme, pine, balsam, and birch are the aromatic essential oils known for their antiseptic properties as well as for their uplifting anti-stress qualities.

The Sagamore Spa utilizes all these exceptional native herbs, flowers, and barks of the mountains and forests that are native to this historic land.

SPAS AROUND THE WORLD

Thalassotherapy Centre, Monte Carlo

This four-level, 6,600-square-meter spa is perched on a cliff overlooking the blue waters of the Mediterranean. The Centre is ideally situated for thalassotherapy—a Greek word meaning "to heal by the sea," using the minerals and microorganisms of seawater to aid in the exchange of impurities from the blood system.

The thalassotherapy program includes 35° C thermal baths, sea mud baths, seaweed treatments, two magnificent azure blue seawater swimming pools, jet streams, countercurrent bath, jet showers, boiling bath seaweed rooms, and balneotherapy.

In 1993, Prince Rainier III asked Dr. Yves Treguer to design "seawater thermal baths of Monte Carlo." Today, the Thalassotherapy Centre, founded by Dr. Yves Treguer, is renowned for its medical program. The Centre offers many health-promoting regimens focusing on particular problems such as nicotine addiction, stress-related ailments, sleeping disorders, menopause, and excess weight.

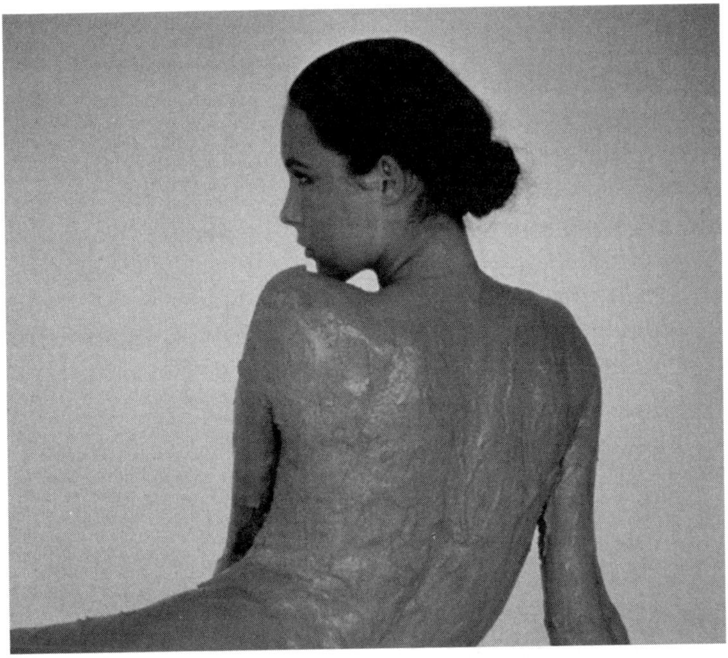

Thalassotherapy Center/Sea Water Thermal Bath of Monte Carlo in the Principality of Monaco. Full body detoxifying treatment with freshly harvested seaweed from the Mediterranean.

All programs focus on the healing, therapeutic virtues of sea elements (seawater, seaweed, sea mud). Seaweed has unquestionable antibiotic, bacteriostatic, and antiviral power. It contains minerals, glucid, proteins, amino acids, vitamins, and phytohormones. Seawater also has the distinction of being "alive" thanks to its microorganisms such as phytoplankton and zoo plankton. When the seawater is heated to around 35° C important chemical exchanges of these elements occur through the skin due to the chemical similarity between blood plasma and seawater. In addition, water is used as a massage element through propelling systems like underwater showers, shower jets, and jet streams.

The water therapy at the Thalassotherapy Centre has healed the physical and mental ailments of countless guests. It certainly would have been endorsed by Euripides, who in 480 B.C. wrote, "The sea heals man's illness."

Termè Di Saturnia Hotel and Spa, Tuscany Regon, Italy

Termè di Saturnia combines "taking the waters" with the opportunity to explore the incredibly beautiful Tuscan countryside of Italy. This spa, complete with its ancient thermal springs, is well known throughout Europe.

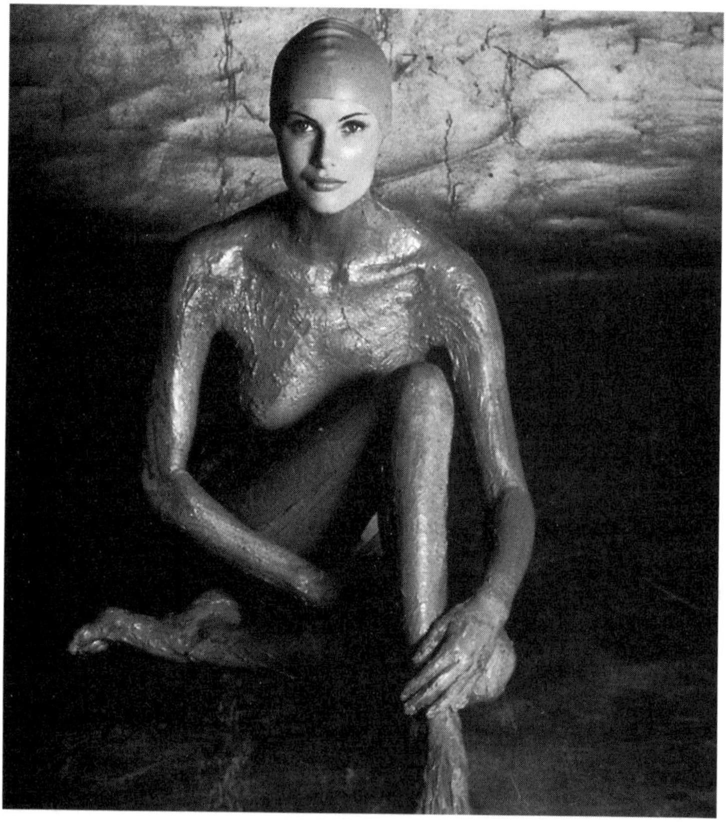

Termè di Saturnia, Tuscany Region, Italy. Special mud treatments from the ancient thermal springs of Saturnia. This thermal mineral mud is used to treat an array of skin problems as well as reduce stress.

Termè di Saturnia, located in the heart of the green rolling hills of Maremma, offers a one-of-a-kind of spa experience. It is unique among all spas because of its 3,000-year-old hot spring that produces 160 gallons of body temperature water every second. Healthful, warm, sulfurous water flows into pools and from waterfalls throughout the spa.

Legend has it that these ancient springs, Saturnia Tellus, were the secret home of the God Saturn. They are also a living memorial to times past when first the Etruscans and then the Romans bathed in their invigorating waters. The Etruscans recognized the therapeutic virtues of the spring and attributed sacred powers to it. The Romans too strongly believed in the healing powers of these warm thermal waters; it was they who turned this site into a spa—a place to rejuvenate and take care of the body. Caesar's legions rested and bathed here. At the end of the seventeenth century the waters of Satunia were recommended as a treatment for skin diseases. The Roman motto for this spa was "Salus Per Aquam," or "Health Through Water." This motto is still appropriate today at the Termè di Saturnia.

The "Skin Enhancing Waters" of Saturnia: Even today, these vigorous springs remain a marvelous natural phenomenon. The secret of the spring water's therapeutic properties is contained in its special composition (sulphuric-carbonic) and its temperature. The rare mineral contents are enriched by their journey through the volcanic subsoil, while the continuous flow of water maintains the crystal purity of the springs. These waters bring direct benefit to many parts of the body, including the respiratory system, muscles, and skin. They are natural medicines that, administered in the appropriate dosage, do not have toxic side effects.

The Therapeutic Mud of Saturnia: The mud of Saturnia is a natural substance produced by the mixture of sulfurous water with organic (algae) and inorganic (minerals) matter that is formed when the clay in hot springs mingles with the thermal waters.

Both the thermal mineral water and the thermal mineral mud of Saturnia are used to treat an array of skin problems: acne, psoriasis, seborrhea, eczema, urticaria, allergic dermatosis. The waters and the mud are also used to help reduce stress.

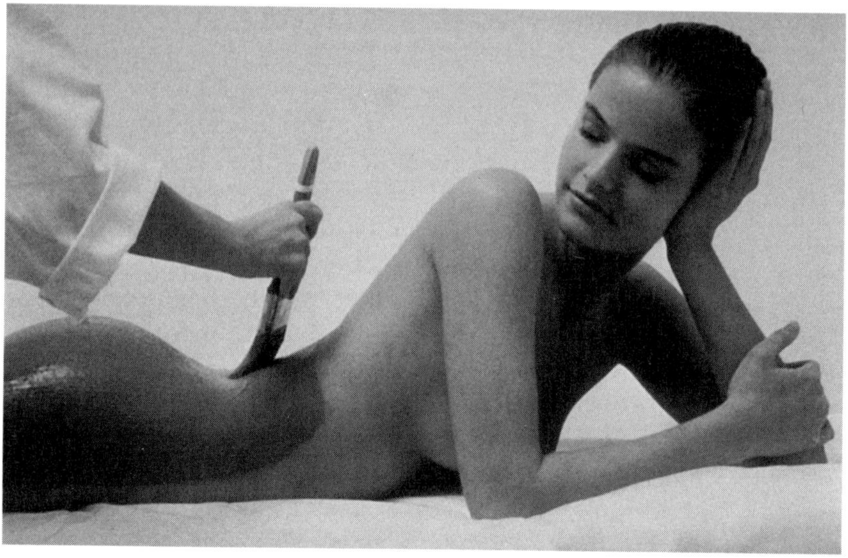

Termè di Saturnia, Tuscany Region, Italy. Special mud treatments from the ancient thermal springs of Saturnia.

Termè di Saturnia offers a wide range of medical and beauty programs. The medical facilities employ five full-time physicians who personalize their testing and treatment plans for each guest. Available beauty and pampering treatments include body toning, anti-stress treatments, facials, skin exfoliation and rehydration, mud masques, and hydromassage.

Moriah Dead Sea Spa, Israel

One of the most spectacular natural phenomena on earth is found in Israel. It is a large salt lake called the Dead Sea. The Moriah Dead Sea Spa sits on the edge of this 47-mile-long body of water that is 1,292 feet below sea level. The River Jordan and a number of tributaries feed into the Dead Sea. Although the sea has no outlets, it never rises more than a few feet due to the high evaporation rate in the desert.

The Dead Sea salt and mineral contents are five times more intense than any ocean. Chlorine, bromine, sodium, sulfate, potassium, calcium, and magnesium are all found in great amounts (the percentage and concentration of these salts and minerals increase the deeper you plunge).

Even though the Dead Sea is absent of fish and almost all organic life, the surrounding area is far from dead. The migration of visitors who want to gain the therapeutic benefits of the water and mud of the Dead Sea keep the area very active. The winter climate is hot and dry and the Dead Sea's therapeutic skin-enhancing properties for skin diseases (especially psoriasis) makes this location a must-see when in Israel.

There are many health and beauty treatments available at the Moriah Dead Sea Spa. A few include:

Indoor Heated Dead Sea Water Pool: Guests feel light as a feather as they float atop the Dead Sea saltwater. The high concentration of health-promoting minerals nourishes the skin and seeps into joints and muscles. The warm (36 degree C), mineral-rich water eases aches and pains and stimulates circulation so guests feel both relaxed and energized. Recommended time in the pool: 15–20 minutes, followed by 15 minutes of rest.

Private Sulfur Bath with Mud: A sulfur bath with Dead Sea mud combines the health-promoting advantages of sulfur with the special skin-enhancing properties of mud. This bath is administered in the privacy of a private bathroom. Recommended time in bath: 15 minutes, followed by 15 minutes rest.

Mud Pack: Black mud is a thick mixture of earth, salts, and organic materials, originating from the Dead Sea floor and then homogenized with water. The warmed mud nourishes the skin, dilates blood vessels, and improves the flow of blood to the skin, muscles, and joints. The mud pack lifts out dirt, grime, and excess grease from pores, while it provides the skin with vital nutrients. The rich concentration of minerals helps to relieve rheumatic pains and promotes a wonderful feeling of cleanliness and relaxation, leaving the skin smooth and toned. Treatment time: 15 minutes.

The Oriental Spa Thai Health and Beauty Center at The Oriental, Bangkok in Thailand

For thousands of years, the ancient practices of the Orient have been revered as the ultimate restorative techniques for both body and soul. Asian methods are renowned for their soothing, healing, and relaxing effects from Shiatsu massage and reflexology to meditation and potent herbal treatments. By combining the Asian philosophy of relaxation and services with a full range of European skin care and body treatments, The Oriental Spa brings a new dimension to the art of rejuvenation. Treatments range from traditional skin care, hydrotherapy, aromatherapy, mud and seaweed body wraps to unique Thai herbal treatments featuring plants and herbs grown especially for the spa by tribes in the northernmost hills of Thailand. The Oriental Body Glow is a good example of one of this spa's unique treatments. A powder scrub made from therapeutic plants grown by the Royal Project in Northern Thailand are blended with essential oils for this gentle exfoliation treatment.

EXOTIC SKIN AND BODY SPA SERVICES

The service menu at a spa is similar to the concept of a menu at a fine restaurant. Even though most restaurants serve pasta, each will serve it in a unique way, giving it a personalized signature style. Below you will find a list of brief descriptions of some of the beauty and massage services you will find at the better spas throughout the world. The exact method of administering these services will vary from place to place, but the basic concept is the same.

Acupressure massage: An ancient, Chinese massage technique used to restore the unrestricted flow of energy by stimulating specific pressure points in the body.

Aerobics: A series of rhythmic exercises, set to music, used to stimulate the aerobic capacity of heart and lungs, and to burn fat.

Aromatherapy: A body massage with fragrant essential oils used for different therapeutic effects.

Aquaerobics: Aerobic exercises in an exercise pool using the support and resistance of the water.

Balneotherapy: The use of waters to restore and revitalize the body. Since antiquity, balneotherapy has been used to improve circulation, fortify the immune system, and reduce pain and stress.

Body composition analysis: A method of measuring the ratio of body fat against lean muscle mass. Used to determine a realistic weight-loss goal and to create a diet and exercise program suited to individual requirements.

Brush and tone: A dry brushing of the skin, intended to remove dead skin cells and impurities while stimulating circulation. This is one of many exfoliating techniques used as a pretreatment for mud and seaweed body masques. A moisturizing lotion completes the treatment, leaving your skin silky smooth, alive and glowing.

Caliper test: A test that determines a person's body fat percentage.

Cathiodermie: A rejuvenating treatment for the skin using low-voltage electrical stimulation. This treatment removes impurities and stimulates regeneration.

Cell therapy: Injections of concentrated live tissue derived from fetal lamb. Administered by physicians in Europe and used to slow the symptoms of aging.

Dancercize: Aerobic workout using steps and patterns of movement derived from modern dance.

Dead Sea mud treatment: Applications of the mineral-rich mud from the Dead Sea in Israel. Used to detoxify skin and body; also used to ease painful symptoms of rheumatism and arthritis.

Dulse scrub: A vigorous body scrub with a mixture of powdered dulse seaweed and oil or water, removing dead skin and providing a mineral and vitamin treatment to the skin.

Electrotherapy: Treatment using the stimulating properties of a low-voltage electrical current.

Fango (the Italian word for mud): A highly mineralized mud mixed with oil or water, warmed, and then applied over the body as a heat pack to detoxify the muscles and stimulate the circulation.

Gommage: A cleansing/exfoliating/rehydrating treatment, using creams that are applied in long, massage-type movements.

Herbal wrap: A body wrap, using strips of cloth that are soaked in heated, herbal solution and wrapped around the body, followed by a period of rest. Used for relaxation as well as to eliminate and detoxify impurities.

Hydrotherapy: Water therapy that includes underwater jet massage, showers, jet sprays, and mineral baths. This therapy has long been a staple in European spas.

Iodine-brine therapy: Mineral baths, naturally rich in salt and iodine, used mostly in Europe for recuperation and convalescence.

Kneipp baths: Herbal/mineral baths. Based on the thermal treatments of Father Sebastian Kneipp, these are highly regarded in Europe.

Loofah scrub: A full-body scrub with a loofah sponge, used to exfoliate the skin and stimulate circulation.

Low-impact aerobics: An aerobic style of exercise that eliminates jumping and other forceful movements to avoid unnecessary injury to the body.

Lymph drainage: A specialized therapeutic massage using a gentle pumping technique to drain away pockets of water retention and trapped toxins. Considered by many European doctors as a premier anti-aging treatment. Lymph drainage can be achieved through manual massage, hydro massage, or with aromatherapy massage.

Moor peat baths: A natural peat preparation, rich in organic matter, proteins, vitamins, and trace minerals, applied to ease aches and pains.

Parafango: Volcanic mud mixed with paraffin wax, often used to treat rheumatism and arthritis.

Paraffin treatment: Heated paraffin wax brushed over the body, trapping heat and drawing out toxins, also promoting relaxation. Treatments leave the skin silky smooth.

Phytotherapy: Healing treatments derived from plants, herbs, aromatic essential oils, seaweeds, and herbal and floral extracts. Applied through massage, packs or wraps, water and steam inhalation, and taken in herbal teas.

Polarity massage: A massage technique developed by Dr. Randolph Stone, used to release pent-up energy through gentle manipulation.

Reflexology: An ancient Chinese technique using pressure-point massage (usually on the feet, but also on the hands and ears) to restore the flow of energy throughout the body.

Repaichage: A treatment applied to the face or full body, using a combination of herbal, seaweed, and clay or mud masks to create deep cleansing and moisturizing.

Rolfing: A massage technique aimed at correcting problems with muscular-skeletal alignment. A series of treatments will move from localized areas where movement is restricted to a structural reorganization of larger body segments. This method of intensive manipulation may sometimes be experienced as painful.

Roman bath: Although the original Roman baths consisted of hot, warm, and cold pools, today the term usually refers to a hot whirlpool/Jacuzzi with benches to sit on.

Salt glow: A body rub with coarse salt, sometimes in combination with fragrant oils, to remove dead skin cells and stimulate circulation.

Sauna: Dry heat in a wooden cabin, used to open the pores and eliminate toxins through perspiration. In combination with refreshing cold showers, saunatherapy helps to relieve stress.

Scotch hose: High-pressure water therapy applied with a hose. The hot and cold fresh or seawater has a massaging action on the skin. This water therapy helps to soothe sore muscles and stimulate circulation.

Seaweed wrap: A highly concentrated mixture of seawater and seaweed that can be called either a wrap or a masque. The ocean's nutrients, minerals, trace elements, and proteins help to revitalize the skin.

Shiatsu: An acupressure massage technique, developed in Japan, applying pressure to specific points in the body to stimulate and open the "meridians" (the pathways in the body through which life energy flows).

Sports massage: Deep-tissue massage, directed specifically at muscles used in athletic activities.

Swiss shower: Powerful shower jets, directed at the body from various heights, creating the effect of an invigorating massage.

Thalassotherapy: Treatments using the therapeutic benefits of the sea and seawater products. Includes seaweed and algae wraps, and also seawater hydrotherapy.

Vichy shower: A shower from several overhead jets, while lying on a waterproof, cushioned mat. This treatment is often followed by exfoliating treatments such as dulse scrub, loofah, or salt-glow.

Wassertanzen (pronounced Vasser-tahn-sen): Underwater choreographed dance.

Watsu: Short for "Water Shiatsu," a kind of underwater, passive yoga.

Waxing: The removal of unwanted hair from face, arms, legs, or body, using soft or hard wax.

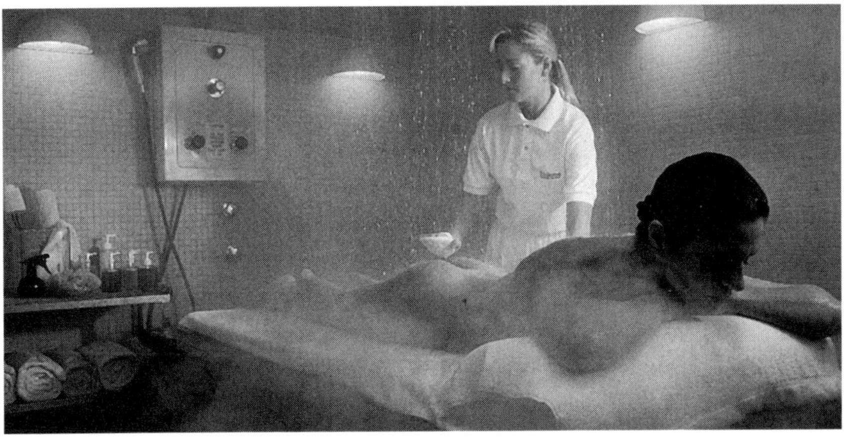

The Spa International at Fisher Island Club, Fisher Island, Florida. Guest enjoying a Vichy shower. This therapeutic spa treatment has several overhead jets and is administered while lying on a waterproof cushioned mat. An exfoliating treatment such as either a salt-glow, loofah scrub, or dulse scrub follows the Vichy shower.

SUM IT UP!

The world of professional spas is quite extensive—we have touched just the surface of this vast industry. But from these brief peeks, you should now have an inkling into what therapeutic and body-pampering treatments await you around the world. You can choose your spa based on the healing and rejuvenating resources of the region: the seaweed and seawater from the ocean; the mineral salts and mineralized sand from the deserts; the thermal mineral waters and muds scattered about the globe, unique regional plants and foods, and even fresh rainwater collected from deserts before it touches the earth.

From the beginning of time, the best beautifying treatments have come from Mother Nature, and they are still healing body and mind today. Don't you think it's about time you experienced a skin-enhancing and stress-reducing spa adventure?

CHAPTER

Fourteen

DISCOVER THE TRADE SECRETS OF LEADING ESTHETICIANS AND SPA EXPERTS

Estheticians and spa experts have more to give their clients than just the spa/salon treatments. Each client who visits a skin expert is sent home with plenty of valuable advice he or she can use every day to maintain the health and appearance of the skin. Estheticians know home care is important because even if you do have regular facials (every four to six weeks), what happens to your skin the rest of the time can either enhance your complexion or destroy it. For this chapter I have interviewed a group of skin experts and asked them to tell us their trade secrets so you can try them at home. The result of these interviews is some very valuable information that you can incorporate into your schedule 365 days a year.

DON'T WASTE TIME!—SKIN CARE YOU CAN DO IN ONE MINUTE

How can I take care of my skin when I have absolutely no time for anything complicated?

"Most people seem to have a problem with time and say they can't take care of their skin," states Robin Kluge, spa director for Maximus Salon and Day Spa in Merrick, New York. "But I've found a simple trick that works for most people on a tight schedule: Keep your cleanser in the shower." Just squeeze out some cleanser and clean your face while in the shower; this takes care of your cleansing needs. When you step out of the shower just splash some toner or water on your face and apply your moisturizer and you're done.

THREE QUICK FIXES FOR YOUR DELICATE EYES

How do you prevent the eyes from becoming sensitive and irritated when you remove eye makeup?

The eyes are the most sensitive area of the face and they do need special care when removing eye makeup. Pat Warren, esthetician and owner of Faces Unlimited, a skin-care clinic in Portland, Oregon, advises that your eye makeup should be removed with a fragrance- and alcohol-free type of product. And if you wear contact lenses you should not use an oily product because this can leave residue on your contact lenses. A special secret that Pat shares with her clients with sensitive eyes is this: If you are not using the waterproof type of mascara, you can remove your eye makeup with warm water and cotton. Just saturate the cotton pad with water and press it gently against your eyes for a few moments; then gently wipe the area.

When the eyes get stressed-out, bloodshot, and overworked, what remedy will refresh them?

Our eyes suffer a great deal of stress during the day: pollution, pollen, reading, fluorescent lighting, and computers all strain the eyes. No wonder your eyes feel stressed and look bloodshot. What should you do? Esther Feit, spa director for Cappellini's Salon and Day Spa in Woodmere, New York, uses an old Chinese remedy. She suggests moistening two Chinese tea bags with water and placing them in the refrigerator. When chilled, place one tea bag on each eye for 10 minutes or until the tea bag loses its chill. Repeat as often as needed. Your eyes will look and feel more refreshed because Chinese tea has a vasoconstricting (tightening) action so your eyes won't appear to look as irritated after this treatment.

How do you reduce under-eye circles without the use of makeup?

Camouflaging dark under-eye circles is usually accomplished with makeup, but there are a couple of simple steps you can take to help reduce the intensity of this problem naturally. First let's understand where dark circles originate from: Allergies, lack of sleep, skin tone, and the way your eyes are positioned in the eye socket all contribute to this problem. Pat Warren, owner of Faces Unlimited, suggests that when you improve the circulation in this area, you help perk up the complexion, which ultimately helps to minimize the dark under-eye cast. When applying your eye creme, use gentle, upward tapping movements by using the tips of your ring finger and pinkie. Also, if you do not have sensitive skin, Pat suggests that you locate an eye creme with stimulating properties (vasodilators) that will help improve the circulation to this area. Look for these ingredients in these products: horse chestnut, arnica, and lemongrass.

BABY FACE! THREE WAYS TO SOOTHE YOUR SENSITIVE SKIN

My skin is super-sensitive, allergy prone, and extra dry. When I apply fragrance-free skin-care products to my face I feel a mild stinging and slight burning. What am I doing wrong?

Even products that are specially formulated for sensitive and allergy-prone skin can sometimes cause a mild tingling sensation. This happens because you don't have the protection of your skin's natural oil (sebum), which helps to dilute the concentrated ingredients in the product. Your dry skin exacerbates any sensitivities you may have. You can counteract this situation quite simply: All you need to do is premoisten your skin with plenty of water before you cleanse your skin and when you apply your moisturizer. The water will dilute the product, which will make it milder to use on your delicate skin.

After a full week of work my skin looks tired. What can I do to refresh my complexion?

Believe it or not, oxygen can help revive you and your skin. "We all take breathing for granted," states Laurie Hostetler, owner and yoga specialist of the posh Kerr House in Grand Rapids, Ohio. Deep breathing and placing your head lower than your hips is a valuable beauty secret that she shares with all her spa guests. It's simple to do! Laurie advises that you can either lie on the floor and lift your legs or even lie on your bed and hang your head over the side of the bed (depending on your physical condition). This technique helps to reverse and relieve the ever-constant pull of gravity that is tugging at us all the time. Deep breathing is another way to get oxygen to your skin, says Laurie. It is important to get all the used air out of the lungs (it's all waste from your body) so you can use full lung capacity in your deep breathing. Deep breathing positively affects your vitality and your complexion by bringing oxygen-rich blood to the skin cells.

Laurie also offers another quick beauty tip to revive a tired complexion— how about an oatmeal facial for your tired, stressed, and irritated skin? (Some nutritious foods can also be very good for the outside of our skin too.) It's simple to make: Just put 1/2 cup of old-fashioned oatmeal in a blender and process until semi-fine. Then mix with a few tablespoons of yogurt (consistency should be moist, not runny). If your skin is dry you can add 1/3 cup of blended avocado or banana to the mix; the oils in either of these two foods can help replenish the skin.

What is the best "all-natural" way to soothe windburn and sunburn?

If you have sensitive skin and the over-the-counter preparations irritate your skin, here's a safe bit of advice from Kimberly Wright, body and beauty manager for the Nemacolin Woodlands Spa in Farmington, Pennsylvania. Kim suggests using red raspberries. To make a raspberry masque take one cup of berries and crush or mash with a fork. Then apply this mixture to the problem area, covering the windburn or sunburn. Leave on the skin for about 5 to 10 minutes. Then rinse well with cool water. Red raspberries are considered a natural analgesic and will help to reduce redness from the inflammation.

Betty Schneider, esthetician for the Grand Wailea Spa in Wailea, Hawaii, shares an ancient Hawaiian remedy for relieving inflammations. The Ti Leaf (from a bushlike plant native to the Hawaiian islands) helps to soothe, calm, and take the sting out of inflamed skin. Betty suggests you gently crush the leaves in your hand to release the therapeutic fluids. Then place them on your skin for about 10 minutes. This will calm the burned and inflamed area.

ENERGIZE YOUR SKIN! THREE NO-FAIL WAYS TO REFRESH TIRED LOOKING SKIN

What kind of facial massage can I perform on myself to give my face better circulation?

Massage is one of the most beneficial skin-care treatments because it helps to relieve stress and to improve circulation. "The perfect time to massage your skin is when you're applying a facial masque," says Carol Combs, owner of Green Valley Spa & Tennis Resort in St. George, Utah. All the advice that is given at the Green Valley Spa is designed to reduce stress and improve the complexion. Here's a simple "Green Valley Spa Massage" you can try at home.

Place some of your masque in the palm, slide your hands together, spreading the masque over your fingers and thumbs. (The Green Valley Spa freshly mixes a cellulose-based masque with garden vegetables (potato juice) and fruits and resinous plant life such as frankincense, myrrh, and amber, and also combines fragrant nectar of fresh rose blossoms.) Then, gliding your fingers over the skin in an up-and-outward motion, cover your entire décolleté, neck, and face with the masque.

Using your fingertips like little tom-toms dancing over your skin, trace a fluid line over the face to keep the masque in place. Start at the chin with both forefingers and tap in both directions at once, moving up the jawline to the ears. Softly resting your forefingers beside the ears, move your thumbs back down the underside of delicate tissue beneath the jawbone. Now you have molded a firm, taut chin line.

Trace a smile by placing both forefingers just below the lower lip and tap out, up, and in again, surrounding both lips with a moist, curving line. While you are tracing, hold your fingers still for a moment just outside the lip line to make certain the masque has an upturned mouth.

Turn your hands in toward each other. Touching the fingertips together, make a little teepee to rest over the nose, pressing lightly into the side of the bridge with the edge of your forefingers.

Next, trace circles around the eyes. Tapping the forefingers again, circle above the browline and down to the upper edge of the cheekbone. Rest your forefingers there while you make light thumbprints underneath the lower ledge, completing the circle at the nose. Then, make a smaller circle by tapping ever so lightly around the eye socket, coming to rest with both forefingers beside the bridge of the nose.

To soften the lines and ridges along the brow, tap a line with both fingers in a continuous fluid motion, moving together up the center of the forehead to the hairline, out to the edge of the face and back into the center, separating and moving back together, dancing down, in and out, as they cover the brow with a tender, lilting song. Tap in place between the eyebrows for a moment; then hold your fingers closely together as they float down the bridge of the nose.

As a finishing touch, gently tweak the end of the nose between your forefinger and thumb; do this again below the bottom lip and then at the tip of the chin to give the masque a distinguished countenance.

What steps can I take to dry up that occasional blemish?

This nuisance can not only be unsightly but it can also hurt if the blemish becomes inflamed. Here is a quick and simple solution that esthetician Karen Ballou shares with all her clients. Mix one teaspoon of kaolin (Chinese clay, which can be purchased in a health-food store) and 2 drops of peppermint and 2 drops of eucalyptus essential oils and mix well. Apply this mixture directly on the blemish. Leave on overnight and rinse off in the morning. The drying and antiseptic properties of this remedy will keep the blemish from appearing enlarged and inflamed. Ballou also suggests applying one drop of peppermint and one drop of eucalyptus essential oil directly to the pimple. These two essential oils have a cooling effect and will help to subdue the heat generated by the infection. Also, both these oils are extremely antiseptic in nature and will kill bacteria on the surface of the skin.

What cleansing advice would you give someone with red, irritated dry skin?

Cleansing dry skin can be an unpleasant experience if certain precautions aren't taken. Your skin is already in a state of trauma, and you don't need to add insult to injury. The goal is not to strip the skin of precious moisture and oil. Anca Saladie, spa director for the exclusive Nordstrom Day Spa in Paramus, New Jersey, alerts all her dry-skin clients on the pitfalls of harsh cleansing habits: no hot water, no harsh towels, and no soap. Anca suggests applying a mild, fragrance-free milky cleanser to premoistened skin and gently massaging the skin with your fingertips in circular movements. Do your serious cleansing in the evening when you are removing makeup. In the morning, give yourself a light mini-cleansing by simply splashing water on your face or using an alcohol- and fragrance-free toner.

EIGHT HOME REMEDIES THAT WILL CORRECT ANNOYING SKIN PROBLEMS

Is there an "all-natural" beauty treatment (besides AHAs) that can help remove flaky skin from my face?

Pineapples and grapefruits have enzymes that will soften and help to dissolve dead skin cells. Look for skin products (cleansers, moisturizers, peels, and exfolients) that contain either of these fruit enzymes. You might also try this remedy: Mix 1 tablespoon of pineapple or grapefruit juice and pulp with

3 tablespoons of kaolin (Chinese clay) and apply to your face for 10 minutes, then rinse well (avoid eye area). This will also help get rid of flaky, dead skin cells.

What can I do for the skin on the neck and décolleté that's beginning to look like chicken skin?

The neck and the décolleté should be considered part the facial area, but unfortunately they are sometimes neglected. Exposure to the sun and neglect can weather this area, making you look old before your time. "Exfoliating this area can help smooth rough, textured skin," states Kimberly Wright, body and beauty manager of the Nemacolin Woodlands Spa in Farmington, Pennsylvania. One of Kim's exfoliating beauty secrets is using "corncob meal," which can be found in health-food stores. To make this skin-smoothing mixture take two tablespoons of corncob meal and add one teaspoon of wheatgerm oil and mix into a pastelike consistency. Apply to your neck and décolleté and massage gently in upward circular movements. Wipe off mixture, then rinse well. Then apply Kim's hydrating masque that you can make in a minute: Beat one egg white with a tablespoon of honey and one teaspoon of wheatgerm oil. Apply to neck and décolleté and leave on for 5 to 10 minutes. Rinse well and then apply a rich moisturizer.

My face is always ruddy-looking and it feels warm. What can I do to control this problem without using makeup?

There are a number of factors that could cause this condition: hot flashes due to menopause, dilated capillaries, and sensitivities to changes in the weather or spicy foods. Your best temporary relief is a soothing compress of cold water. But for those times when cold water is not enough, try mixing a cup of cold water with a tablespoon of cornstarch. The cornstarch will soothe any stinging and reduce the warm sensation. You can also try applying chilled aloe vera gel or a compress of Chinese tea solution. Both will reduce redness and cool down the skin.

My lips are beginning to look old, and the skin on my lips looks dry. I'm applying moisturizer but it isn't working. What can I do to correct this problem?

Moisturizing is not enough; you have to exfoliate the skin, even on your lips. Either a complexion brush or facial scrub will help to remove unwanted dead skin cells. It is important to exfoliate your skin while it is premoistened with water. Don't forget to include the lip line.

The skin on my hands is cracked. I'm using hand creme but it doesn't seem to be doing the trick. How can I make my hands more presentable?

Do you feel as if your hands need a makeover? Dry and cracked skin on the hands can not only look unsightly but can be uncomfortable. The solution is simple! The skin on the hands becomes callused in places and cracks due to dryness so the first step is to remove the calluses. Buffing or polishing the skin with something abrasive should do the trick. Pumice powder, cornmeal, or fine sugar are abrasive ingredients that won't irritate the skin. Moisten your hand first with water, then apply a thick hand creme. Then take a tablespoonful of one of these abrasive ingredients (either pumice powder, cornmeal, or fine sugar) and begin to massage all over your hands, concentrating on the problem areas. Rinse well, then apply a rich hand creme. You will have to repeat this treatment every other day until the problem is under control.

How can I perk up my dull, devitalized complexion? It looks so pale.

This type of skin can make you look sickly. The dullness can come from either an accumulation of dead skin cells or a sallow skin tone. In either case the way to improve this problem is simple. To remove the accumulation of dead skin cells try exfoliating with a natural-bristle facial brush moistened with water and aloe vera gel. Use a minimal amount of pressure, use small circular movements, and don't forget to avoid the eye area.

Here's another solution for dullness: "After cleansing your skin, apply a warm compress of vitamin C-rich, rosehip tea solution," suggests Kimberly Wright, the body and beauty manager for the Nemacolin Woodlands Spa in Farmington, Pennsylvania. To make the solution, steep two rosehip teabags in boiling water for 15 to 20 minutes. When the water is warm to the touch, saturate a large piece of cotton or an old terry towel (use an *old* towel because the tea will cause a stain). Apply to your face for approximately 5 to 10 minutes. Do not rinse your face after this treatment. You can save the rosehip solution and use it as a facial tonic after cleansing or you can steam your face with the rosehip solution.

The skin on my elbows and knees looks darker and scalier than the rest of my skin. Is there a special treatment I can do at home to correct this unsightly problem?

Thick, callused skin often takes on a dark, almost stainlike appearance on the elbows and knees. This problem can become embarrassing, especially when you want to wear short sleeves and shorts. Moisturizing the skin is not adequate because it does not remove the dead, callused skin. The remedy for this problem can be found in your kitchen. Take one cup of cornmeal, mix it with a 1/3 cup of fresh lemon or lime juice and 2 tablespoons of aloe vera gel. Massage your elbows and knees with this mixture. Repeat this treatment every other day until you see improvement. Remember, this problem did not happen overnight.

My complexion looks so uneven. What can I do?

An ancient remedy for this problem is "rice water," which has been used for thousands of years by the women of China. When the rice was harvested, they soaked it in rainwater. Then the rice water was saved and used as a facial tonic because it was believed to have skin-lightening properties. In some provinces of China they ground the rice into an extra-fine dustlike texture and used it as a face powder. You can make your own rice water at home. Put a few cups of rice in a colander. Place the colander into a large bowl of water and let the rice soak for about one hour. Lift the colander and rice out of the bowl; the remaining water is your facial tonic for uneven skin tone.

GET RID OF STRESS IN FIVE EASY STEPS

I need to relax, but I don't have the time. Are there quick relaxation tips I could use when I'm stressed-out at work or at home?

Stress can take its toll on your energy level and ultimately your complexion. Renee Rauch, R.D., life enhancement manager for the Spa at Doral in Miami, Florida, takes the business of reducing stress very seriously. Renee offers five quick and simple solutions that will soothe even the most frazzled nerves.

1. Relax your eyes. To relax your eyes is to relax your whole body. Because so much of our sensory imput is visual, temporarily closing off this channel will almost immediately cause the rest of the body to slow down. Brain-wave patterns change to a lower frequency as soon as the eyes are closed. Resting your eyes is an important way of reestablishing balance throughout the system and reducing unnecessary strain.
   - Sit or lie down and take a few moments to breathe deeply.
   - Gently close your eyes.
   - Place the palms of your hands over your eyes.
   - Use memory and imagination to realize a perfect black field.
   - Do not try to produce any experience. Simply allow the blackness to happen. Continue for two to three minutes, breathing easily.
   - Remove your hands from your eyes and open your eyes slowly.
   - Do this whenever you feel you need to relax.
2. Warm your hands for relaxation. By relaxing and focusing on warming your hands you can raise your hand temperature as much as 20 degrees F in five minutes. The result of hand warming is usually a deep state of relaxing, or one of the altered states of consciousness experienced in meditation. It helps the body to carry out its self-repair. Here's how to do it:
   - Sit in a relaxed position.
   - Place your hands on your lap, palms facing up, fingers relaxed.
   - Slowly begin to say to yourself, "My hands are getting warmer."
   - Repeat this several times.

- Combine the repetition of the words with a mental picture that suggests warm hands.
- See your hands being bathed in warm water, or holding your hands up to the sun, and so on.
- In your mind's eye surround your hands with a glowing warm light.
- Feel your hands getting warmer.

3. Candle mediation. Light a candle in a semi-darkened room. Place it about 20 inches from you at eye level. Look at it. Become absorbed in it.
   - As thoughts arise bring your attention back to the awareness of the candle and flame.
   - Try not to mentally analyze or describe what is taking place. Simply be with it.
   - Close your eyes and find the images imprinted on your eyelids. Stay with it.
   - As it fades, open your eyes and see the candle again.
   - Do this for 10 minutes.
4. Breathing exercise. Try this exercise sitting, standing or lying down.
   - Exhale deeply, contracting the abdomen.
   - Inhale slowly as you expand the abdomen.
   - Continue inhaling as you raise the shoulders up toward your ears.
   - Hold for a few comfortable seconds.
   - Exhale in reverse pattern, slowly. Release shoulders, relax chest, contract the abdomen.
   - Repeat.
5. Hot toddy recipe. Make yourself a hot apple toddy. Elevate your feet, relax, and enjoy. Ingredients: 1 cup nonfat milk, 1 cup applesauce, 1/4 ground cinnamon, 1/2 teaspoon vanilla extract. Blend until smooth. Serve hot in your favorite mug and garnish with cinnamon sticks.

Are there any relaxation techniques that will calm my fidgety infant?

Even infants can get stressed out. "Infant massage therapy helps to relieve stress," says Karen Ballou, esthetician and owner of Babyderm in Bolingbrook, Illinois. Massage is a nonverbal communication that builds a loving bond between parent and child. Karen says the perfect time for the massage is after a bath when the baby is beginning to relax. Here are a few quick tips on the massage technique.

- Create a quiet time for the you and the baby.
- Have soft music nearby that the baby will eventually learn to associate with her relaxing massage time.
- Begin the massage on a comfortable surface.
- Take a deep breath and relax a few moments before you begin the massage.
- Not much product is needed; just a small amount of a lightweight, nongreasy moisturizer is used throughout the massage.
- Have a blanket ready for the baby when done. He needs to be kept warm.
- Warm up the lotion in your hands before you begin.
- Place your baby on her back and begin your massage at her feet.
- Use light, flowing movements while working upward. (The baby may move around at first; give him a toy he can look at and hold if necessary.)
- Turn the baby on her stomach when you finish with the back.
- Remember, babies move a lot. Be patient as he becomes familiar with the new sensations.
- When the baby is on her stomach, begin again at the ankles or feet with light, flowing upward movements.
- Don't show the baby any frustration on your part or you will send an unpleasant message.
- If the baby is unable to lie quietly through a whole massage, do as much as you can and stop. Each time you do a massage, you will find you can do a little more.

- You may want to keep a diaper on the baby during your massage and remove it somewhat when you massage the buttocks.
- When you finish, don't remove the moisturizer; begin to dress the baby. This would be a good time for bedtime or a nap.

This nurturing touch helps the baby relax and relieve the stresses that build up daily from so many new encounters with the world.

BACK TO BASICS SKIN CARE

I get so confused when I look at all the products in the stores that I end up buying nothing. What can I do?

Laura Hittleman, head esthetician for the Canyon Ranch Spa in Lenox, Massachusetts, believes in the "getting back to the basics" concept. Begin with one good cleansing and moisturizing product that you can use every morning and night. Also, Laura suggests that you're never too young to use an eye creme because this is such a neglected area as well as a delicate zone of the face.

How can I calm myself from a stressful day?

Robin Russell, skin care therapist and consultant relies heavily on the power of essential oils. Ms. Russell suggests locating a pre-blended calming essential oil and combine 5 to 10 drops of this oil with 1/2 cup of warm water in a small bowl. Quickly place a washcloth into the bowl while the water is still warm and allow it to absorb essential oil mixture. Then wring out excess fluid and place washcloth on the back of your neck. Place the palms of your hands together and rub to form friction. With the warmth from your hands place palms on your closed eyelids and relax for a couple of minutes.

SUM IT UP!

So the secrets are out! There certainly are many at-home, skin-care regimens that use inexpensive, natural ingredients to help correct or reduce skin problems. These professionals have tried and proven their effectiveness and now offer them to you. If you would like more personalized skin-care advice, be sure to contact an esthetician or spa expert and schedule an appointment. If you're not sure where to find a qualified skin expert, there are national esthetic organizations that can help you find one in your area (see Appendix A on page 355). But between visits, keep your skin healthy and attractive with the secrets you've learned here.

APPENDIX A

THE ABCs OF YOUR SKIN-CARE PRODUCTS

The increasingly fast pace of the skin-care industry has made it difficult to truly understand the function of many of the new products available. What was a rather uncomplicated visit to the salon, department store, or drug store to select a cleanser or moisturizer is now much more complicated due to the vast selections.

Selecting the correct product during any life stage could be challenging because all products are not created equal. A product usually focuses on a particular skin type (acne, oily, normal, dry) or condition (mature, sun-damaged, sensitive). For example a product for acne, oily, and normal skin would not help a mature or sun-damaged skin in its quest for moisture. In fact these types of products for oily or acne skin would actually rob moisture from a dry skin type because they are usually oil-free. It is the oil content plus the humectant (ingredient that attracts moisture to the skin) that help dry skin retain precious moisture.

The type of ingredients that are used in a formula will dictate the efficacy of its performance and whether a product is appropriate for your skin or not. Chemists spend years in matching skin enhancing active ingredients to address the needs of your skin.

The following information will help you discover the meaning for the terms used by the skin-care industry as well as focus on a few of the ingredients used to help maintain a youthful appearance.

Terms You Should Know About Your Skin-care Product

Alcohol-Free: Alcohol-free means that the product does not contain certain alcohols (for instance, SD alcohol). It may contain alcohol such as cetyl alcohol, which is an ingredient used as an emulsifying agent in cremes and which does not adversely affect certain skin types. Alcohol-free products are especially recommended for individuals with sensitive, dry, and sun-damaged skin.

Free-Radical Scavengers: These are ingredients such as vitamin E (D-alpha-tocopherol, DL-alpha-tocopherol), ginkgo biloba, and super-oxide dismutase. These ingredients help guard the cellular membrane against free radicals created by such things as exposure to the sun, pollution, cigarettes, and eating fried foods.

Fragrance-Free: Fragrances are scents that are added to products to make them have a pleasant odor. However, consumers should be aware that fragrances are the greatest sensitizing ingredient, in other words, they are the ingredient that would most likely cause a possible allergic reaction that might result in a breakout, itching, hives, or irritation. Many manufacturers today are using essential oils to naturally fragrance a skin-care product. These types of oils are more compatible with the skin than a synthetic fragrance.

Hypoallergenic: This term means that the ingredients in the products have been tested for adverse reaction. Only ingredients with a track record of low sensitivity occurrences are used in this type of formula. Products of this nature are usually fragrance- and alcohol-free. If you are extremely sensitive, it is always best to do a patch test of a product on a small area of skin (jawline or behind your ear) and wait 24 hours. If you do not show any sensitivities within that time frame, more than likely your skin is compatible with the product.

Ingredients that Will Help Your Skin Retain Its Youthful Glow

One of the present preoccupations of cosmetic chemists is to create a skin-care formulation able to slow down the aging process. They are turning to new types of ingredients to address the natural aging process of the skin as well as the premature aging due to sun damage. Here are a few ingredients you should keep your eye on.

Sunscreens: This is probably the best antiaging ingredient there is because by using a sunscreen you are protecting your skin from the sun which happens to cause 90% of premature aging (wrinkles, fine lines, age spots, loss of tone). Sunscreens are being added to many products because of their protective nature and their ability to help the skin repair itself. When purchasing this type of product it is important to look for which is called the SPF (Sun Protection Factor). The American Academy of Dermatology recommends that you use no less than a 15 SPF. (For more information on sunscreens and the sun see Chapter Ten: Tanning! The Good and Bad.)

Vitamin C: Our body does not synthesize vitamin C. This important vitamin is an influential antioxidant as well as a major player when it comes to the synthesis of collagen. Topical vitamin C is now being introduced into a few skin-care products. Researchers at Duke University Medical Center, Durham, NC, have developed a stable aqueous formulation of vitamin C (ascorbic acid). That is not only broad-spectrum photoprotective when applied topically but has anti-inflammatory properties and reportedly can work at full force within three days.

Lipids: This substance includes fats, waxes, phosphatides, cerebrosides. When lipids are applied to the skin they have a moisturizing and skin-smoothing action.

Liposomes: Liposomes are microscopic vesicles composed of membrane-like layers separated by an aqueous layer with a fluid center. One of the main functions is to encapsulate an active ingredient. Liposomes provide prolonged release of an active ingredient.

It is cosmetically more acceptable because it provides a less tacky and greasy product.

Alpha Hydroxy Acids: Alpha hydroxy Acids are acids that are either naturally derived from sugar cane or fruits. Best known among them is glycolic acid. All are used for their ability to exfoliate and thus regenerate the skin.

Essential Fatty Acids: Linoleic and linolenic acids cannot be manufactured by the body and must be supplied by a food source. If you are deficient of essential fatty acids it could cause eczema, inflammations of the skin, and scaling. Essential fatty acids are used in moisturizers to help counteract rough, dry, scaly skin.

APPENDIX B

SOURCES OF INFORMATION FOR YOUR SKIN

Esthetic Alternatives®, Inc.
Lynn Parentini
P.O. Box 2525
Fairlawn, NJ 07410
Publishes a bi-yearly educational bulletin about the skin.

American Academy of Dermatology
930 North Meachman Rd.
Schaumburg, IL 60173

American Academy of Cosmetic Surgery
401 Michigan Avenue
Chicago, IL 60611-4267
1 (800) A New You

American Society of Esthetic Medicine, Inc.
5415 N. Sheridan Road
Suite 3210
Chicago, IL 60640-1954
(312) 334-2494
Fax: (312) 334-2290

Skin Cancer Society
245 Fifth Avenue
New York, NY 10016

American Cancer Society
1599 Clifton Road N.E.
Atlanta, GA 30329

National Vitiligo Foundation
P.O. Box 6337
Tyler TX 75711

National Psoriasis Foundation
6443 S.W. Beaverton Hwy.
Suite 210
Portland OR 97221

Eczema Association for Science and Education
1221 S.W. Yarnhill, Suite 303
Portland, OR 97205

The Spa-Finder
91 Fifth Avenue, Suite 301
New York, NY 10003-3039

Index

A

B

C

D

E

F

G

H

N

O

T